The System for Soul Memory

The System for Soul Memory

Using the Energy System of Your Body to Change Your Life

SUSAN KERR

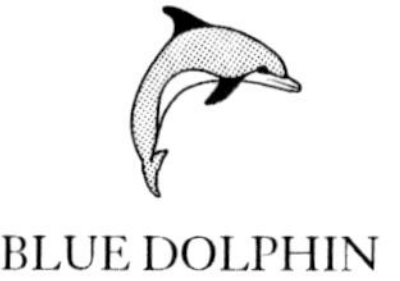

BLUE DOLPHIN

Published by Blue Dolphin Publishing, Inc.
P.O. Box 8, Nevada City, CA 95959
Web : www.bluedolphinpublishing.com
Orders: 1-800-643-0765

ISBN: 1-57733-089-7

Library of Congress Cataloging-in-Publication Data

Kerr, Susan, 1949-
The system for soul memory : using the energy system of your body to change your life / Susan Kerr.
p. cm.
Includes bibliographical references.
ISBN 1-57733-089-7
1. Chakras. 2. Emotions—Psychic aspects. I. Title.

BF1442.C53 K47 2001
1331—dc21

2001035604

Printed in the United States of America

10 9 8 7 6 5 4 3 2 1

Dedication

To Michael,
Joshua, and Zachary,
Who taught me earthly love.

To Mafu,
Who taught me divine love.

Contents

Acknowledgments

I began studying with Mafu and his channel, Paramananda Saraswatti, in 1988. I found Mafu's teachings to be so profound, I began living what I learned. This led to my developing the System for Soul Memory. Therefore, it is hard for me to distinguish what should be actual quotations from Mafu. and what later devolved into my own experiences. That is why with profound love and respect, I acknowledge Mafu's participation in the production of this book, and why a portion of the profits will be given to the Foundation for Meditative Studies.

If you would like to hear Mafu's wisdom in its purity, you can contact:

The Foundation for Meditative Studies
P.O. Box 458
Eagle Point, Oregon 97524

Introduction

Author's History: The Creation of the System for Soul Memory

My whole life has been directed to writing this book. From the moment I was born, my psychic experiences all pointed to this direction. I didn't know this until much later, since so many of the events seemed random and unrelated. During the last ten years everything started coming together. I learned that our life's experiences are no accident. There is a divine plan at work. It wasn't until I could tap into my subconscious, that I could see this more clearly.

The subconscious remembers everything, and through meditation and regression it can be recalled. Because of this, I was able to remember much of my early years. I was surprised at what I discovered, at how differently my subconscious remembered things. That is why, in re-experiencing my birth, I was surprised at what my subconscious recalled. My memories weren't about me, about what it felt like to be born in a cold delivery room with the bright lights and the frenzy of the nurses and doctors; instead my awareness was centered on the people in the room; *on their emotional pain*. I was amazed at discovering this. But from what I know now about my psychic abilities, it all made sense. From the moment I was born, I could feel the emotions of others. Not the easy emotions like happiness and joy, but the deep buried ones most people chose to ignore.

Because of this psychic ability, the world in those early years was a confusing place. The picture of life looked right, but many times it did not feel right. People would approach me with happy faces, but on the inside I knew they were sad. Early on, I became a people pleaser. I wanted to ease their sorrow, help them feel better. I didn't know I was being telepathic. But reading their thoughts and feelings, I was very good at satisfying their needs. They didn't need to be expressed; I could feel them. It wasn't until I became an adult that I began to understand the confusion and make the distinctions.

I also experienced other types of psychic abilities. These taught me that the world existed on many different levels. I remember having incredible dreams. Dreams of events that would later come true, and dreams filled with 'Beings of Light.' These spiritual masters would appear before me filled with love. They would instruct me and tell me tell me things that didn't mean much then, but later would have special significance.

I remember astral traveling, being able to leave my body while in a very relaxed state. Many times as a very young child I would go to bed, then stare down at myself from the corner of the room.

But what I remember most vividly was something that was very scary to me as a little child. I would suddenly awaken from a deep sleep, throbbing with energy. I felt like I was being plugged into an electric socket. The sound was deafening and I always found myself spinning through a dark tunnel to a distant light. The feeling was that I would die if I continued. I learned to stop the rush of energy. (I later learned that people who have lived through near-death experiences have expressed the same sort of sensations.)

In those early years, I had many psychic experiences and no one to explain them to me. Not my parents, or my religion. In fact

I learned early to keep my experiences quiet. I didn't want people thinking I was weird, and I didn't want to frighten them. I also learned to bury my emotions. I didn't want to feel all the misery around me.

When I was seventeen, my mother began a slow process of dying with lung cancer. It was during this time that we both opened up more about psychic phenomena. We talked about reincarnation and heaven. She bought a book, *Edgar Cayce, the Sleeping Prophet,* which told the story of a psychic healer who healed thousands while in a deep, sleep-like, trance.

Reading about him awakened me to a whole new, world. I finally found someone who could explain some of my own experiences. I read every Edgar Cayce book I could find. I turned to metaphysics and found others who had similar experiences. I was finally beginning to understand.

I went to college, got married and had kids, and kept much of my psychic experiences quiet and as shut down as possible. But I did read as many metaphysical books as I could. The dreams with the Beings of Light still continued, only more frequently. So did visions of the future. I saw a new world coming. A spiritual world where everyone walked liked Jesus and Buddha, with love and peace in their hearts. It was like the Garden of Eden returned, where there was no more sickness or war, where everyone could create what they wanted just by thinking about it. But before this world would manifest, there would be many changes and disasters. I saw the earth in upheaval with floods, tidal waves, earthquakes, volcanic eruptions, and terrible storms. I saw large cities in distress, religious wars, and gangs of youths so terrorizing, that curfews were strongly enforced by the militia. I saw the ozone layer being destroyed, causing the sun to become deadly. This forced people to seek refuge underground to escape the harsh rays and the extreme heat. I saw thousands of children dying; lying ill in gymnasiums because there were so many, hospitals could no longer hold them. Some of the visions have already come to pass. I am hoping the bleaker ones can still be changed.

And then in 1987 I met my teacher. His name was Mafu, and a woman, Swami Paramananda Saraswatti, channeled him. Channeling is a psychic phenomenon where a human becomes a vehicle to transfer thought from someone in the spirit world. This practice has been going on for centuries. Even prophets did it in the Bible.

Naturally I would be attracted to an unseen spiritual teacher. They have been around me my whole life coming through to me as the 'Beings of Light.' Mafu had the same feeling of incredible love about him. I recognized him as being one of those 'Beings of Light.' He knew everything about me: my life experiences, my thoughts and my most innermost feelings. In his presence I witnessed miracles, and with his help I finally learned how to accept myself and my psychic abilities. I also learned how to use them to help others. Much of what I learned from him became the foundation of this book. He explained to me what I was experiencing and how it related in more mundane psychological terms.

It was after this that I came out of the 'closet' and announced to the people in my world that I was psychic, that I was 'different'. I opened a metaphysical bookstore, driven by my strong feeling to help others prepare for the new world coming. I started doing spiritual counseling. During these counseling sessions, I too began channeling. Much of the information I received became the basis of this book. It dealt with the soul, the chakras, and the energy system of the body. I began meditating on a daily basis. I was flooded with information. This information always proved useful and accurate.

I continued to have out of body experiences, only this time they were more incredible because they were happening in my meditations. I experienced them as lucid dreams. Some times I meditated and found myself talking to someone who was a total stranger. In the meditation, this person told me his name and what was happening in his life. A few days later, I would actually meet him. Before he could say anything, I would tell him his name, then repeat to him what he had told me days before. Naturally, people were amazed because I would be right. I was always humbled by these experiences.

Meditation began proving to me how we create our future. Whenever I saw future events in my meditations, I knew what to expect. They always proved true.

I also continued to have those episodic surges of energy. I still had no control over them. They happened on their own, either in meditation or sleep. And they all still happened in the same manner, as if an electric switch had been turned on in my body.

The most startling one happened just before I met Mafu. My family and I went to Puerto Rico on vacation. One night I awoke with a start when the 'switch' suddenly turned on. The energy was much more intense than usual. This time I felt my body breaking away from itself. The only way I can explain it is that I became two bodies, my physical one and my spiritual one, which hummed on top of my body like pure electricity. I heard a voice warn me not to touch my husband that I could hurt him if I did. The way I felt, I didn't doubt this for a minute. I looked at him and slid as far to the edge of the bed as possible.

I closed my eyes and gave into the energy as the roaring noise got louder and louder. And then the most incredible thing happened. I started rushing toward the light only this time I experienced the rushing in a very physical way that I could comprehend. I understood exactly what was happening. The light I was rushing towards wasn't scary anymore. It was a light behind my eyes. Once I reached this light I was sucked back into my chest, into my soul. My whole being felt crushed, like it was being compressed. Suddenly, I imploded, and was thrown out of my body through an opening at the back of my neck. Like sweet, caressing nectar, I felt my spirit pour over my head and down the rest of my body.

I began rising like air and leaving the room. As I ventured one last glance at the bed, instead of seeing my husband and myself, I saw two orbs of glowing golden-white light in the general area of our chests.

The next part of the experience was incredible. I found myself in what I can only describe as an expanded state of mind. Everything was black and what I was shown, I witnessed as a hologram. Every thought felt as if it were 'implanted' in my mind. I was shown a heaven, a *pulsating* river of golden stars. I 'knew' this was God. I knew that I, and everyone else, was one of those stars. We are each an atom in God's body—each feeling autonomous and separate, yet really part of the whole. And immediately attached to that knowing came the thought, that every evening, God gives us the night sky to remind us of this.

Then I was shown a hologram of what happens at this level when I do something in the physical. For example if I were to walk down the street, at this level it would be me as a golden light intercepting and moving through millions of other golden lights. In other words, me walking down the street is in mutual agreement with millions of other lights; other parts of God, that have allowed me to use them to create my 'scene' in third dimension of me walking down the street.

The last hologram showed me what happens in God's kingdom when two souls unite in love. It felt like an explosion of ecstasy and it reacted like a wave, eddying through the entire river of golden lights, affecting and expanding all. I was shown how one person loving, affects all of us.

With a jolt of physical awareness, I found myself squeezing back into my body. After feeling so expanded, I couldn't believe how little my body felt. The first thing I did was look at my hand. But I couldn't see it. All I saw were those pulsating golden lights. Like atoms. I stared beyond, at what should have been the wall, but it too was nothing but pulsating golden lights. The roaring was still loud in my ears and the energy still intense. I waited, and within minutes, the roaring began to subside and the energy to quiet. I began to see the wall take shape, the golden lights converging into a mass. Everything was still pulsating.

Needless to say, it took me days to recover, and years to fully understand what took place. When I learned more about Eastern philosophies, I learned about the chakras and the energy system of the body. The light behind my eyes came from my Crown Chakra. The chakra on the back of my neck, where I left my body is called the Moon Center Chakra. (I find it very interesting that when most people experience ghosts and spirits, the hair at the back of the neck rises.) I also learned that those energy surges I experienced my whole life are called the rising of the Kundalini. Many meditators, such as gurus, swamis, and enlightened beings, have written about it. Everyone experiences them on some level.

Once I made it okay to be psychic, I became even more psychic. During a seminar in Oregon, Swami Paramananda Saraswatti taught me a technique to talk to animals. I never thought to use the technique until one day a woman walked into my bookstore with a sad, sick parrot on her shoulder. She adopted it two months before, and she was at her wit's end. The vet could find no physical basis for the bird's failing to eat and talk. She didn't know what to do. The bird was fine when she got it. Now she knew the bird was dying.

It was so easy speaking to her bird that day, the mental images passed easily between us. When I told her that all she had to do was move the bird's cage to a window that he missed seeing the trees outside, she laughed. That's it? She was very skeptical.

But in talking with that bird I had become one with him. Besides the mental images, I felt all the bird's feelings, and through the bird, the woman's feelings too. I saw again God's incredible creation, the oneness of everything despite the fact that it all looks separate. I saw how like energy attracts like energy. The woman attracted the bird into her life to heal an old emotional childhood wound. The bird suffered the same wound in his short life. Through healing the bird, the woman would heal herself; and she wouldn't even know it.

She called me the next day, ecstatic. After spending part of the night rearranging the furniture in her small apartment, she was able to move the cage to the window. As soon as the parrot saw the sun come up he started to squawk and eat. She was amazed. He was a new bird. He was happy and so was she.

She was also the president of a local bird club. So word quickly spread and soon I was speaking to clubs and getting calls to help other animals in distress. Before I knew it, a producer from the Joan Rivers television show called and asked me to be on her show as an animal psychic. After that came the Ricki Lake show, then the Carnie Wilson show. For someone who was a closet psychic and didn't want to be known as weird, I was now known as a 'weirdo' in a major way!

One of the hardest things as a psychic for me to overcome is making it okay to 'scare' people. Being used as a messenger for spirit and passing on psychic information frightens many people. I am always daunted by it, never knowing how people will react. Plus, feeling their emotions is never easy. It is hard going up to a total stranger and relaying to them the psychic message spirit is sending me. Yet, spirit can be so insistent if I protest.

The first time it happened was many years ago and it came in the form of a lucid dream. In the dream I was speaking to a man. He had lesions on his face and he was wearing a scarf around his neck to hide some of them. I knew he was dying of AIDS. In the dream, Jesus appeared and stood behind him. I put my hand on the man's forehead as Jesus instructed, and told him not to worry, Jesus was with him. I then awoke, not surprised by the content of the dream. I knew it was an omen of the future.

Three days later I was travelling on a train to New York City when I spotted the man. He sat two rows up from me. He had lesions on his face and was wearing the same scarf I had seen in the dream. I knew I was supposed to go up to him and relay the message that Jesus was with him and not to worry, but at that time, I couldn't. I wasn't out of the closet yet, and I still had not learned the special significance of those messages to the ones intended.

Afterwards, the experience haunted me. It was a great learning lesson. How many times does a nice Jewish girl see Jesus in her dreams? Yes the man probably would have freaked out and thought me psychotic, but today I know he would have received much comfort from what I could have said. Later thinking about it, I realized that I was judging God's plan for me. I was psychic for a reason.

Now I look back and see how the results from those encounters led me to understanding the soul better. Each time I relayed a message, I learned more about emotions, where they sat in each chakra, and their connection to the soul.

This connection with spirit also led me to understanding the feeling of 'grace.' Opening myself up to accepting messages also opens me up to receiving spirit's love. That feeling of love gives me a great sense of peace and the feeling of being connected with all of life, the seen and unseen. Through receiving the love and messages of others who passed on, I could feel God around me and within me.

It was Mafu who taught me that behind every illness and injury is a buried emotion. It wasn't until a particular meditation that I experienced this for myself. I was spending the week in Oregon, at a special retreat. It was morning and we were all meditating. Suddenly in my meditation, I saw a man. I knew who he was. He was a participant at the retreat, but I didn't know him personally. In the meditation, he showed me his thumb. It was injured. A large V-shaped wedge had been torn out of the nail bed. It was bleeding. At that moment, I came out of the meditation thinking this very strange. When the session was over, I looked for him. I told him what I had seen in my meditation. He blanched and said, "You mean this?" He showed me his thumb. The nail had been torn out just as I had seen it. Only now it was healed. "It happened ten years ago," he went on to say. "What do you think it means?"

"I don't know," I replied. But as he walked away, I knew. In a rush of emotions, I felt a strong surge of abandonment. I knew a woman was the cause, and that he wasn't feeling it. I knew he could re-injure his thumb if he didn't feel the emotion now. Three months later I was talking to his wife and she explained. Ten years before they were having marital problems and she was going to leave him. That's when he injured his thumb. Fortunately they worked it out. But the week of the retreat, she had to leave again. She had to go out of town and couldn't be with him. Apparently he was feeling abandoned again, but instead of feeling the emotion, he was going to cause physical injury to himself.

Afterwards, I experienced this repeatedly. This is the psychic ability I knew as a child, but because it was so overwhelming, I shut it down. Opening the door, allowing it to happen again, was still overwhelming and frightening.

A week later a man was injured while doing outside repair work to the business next door. He tore the skin off his shin in a long gash that later I heard required 22 stitches. For me, his accident was an explosion of emotion. I could feel his misery, misery from an alcoholic and abusive father who beat him as a child. Now he had a boss who was just as abusive. Only he didn't need someone to beat him anymore, he had learned very nicely from his childhood how to do it to himself. A week later I spoke to a fellow worker who confirmed my impressions.

In the beginning, other psychic friends discouraged me from opening myself up so much to others. It's bad they warned. I tried listening to them. I tried shutting myself off to those flooding sensations. But I found I couldn't. It was like cutting off the energy to my body, to who I was. I got physically weak and felt drained if I stopped the flow. Amazingly, if I allowed the emotions of others to pour through me, I felt more energized. The only time the energy got stuck was when I had a personal issue with that emotion too. I found that guilt, rationalization, or self-judgement stopped the flow of energy.

That is when I made it okay to be me. I began making a concerted effort to study energy and the emotions. I began noticing patterns. Emotions are energy that wants to be acknowledged. They don't care who acknowledges them. If I felt someone else's emotions, it was like they were feeling them too. My acknowledging them opened the doorway for them to acknowledge them. I began noticing where the emotions sat in the body. I began learning everything about them. I learned that brain matter doesn't just reside in the brain. It's found down our spine where the chakra's, our energy centers, are found. I learned that our subconscious doesn't reside in our brain. It resides throughout our body. That is what this book is about.

My meditations progressed too. I no longer flew to Oregon to study with Swamiji and Mafu. I could study with them in my meditations. Friends would go to the retreats and when they returned, I would tell them what happened before they could even get it out of their mouths. I learned that besides having a physical body, we have a spirit body too. Metaphysical people call this the astral body, or the dream body. This is the part of you that leaves your body at night when you go to sleep, and permanently when you die. Astral traveling in a meditation is no different than having a lucid dream.

Sometimes at night when my sons would just go off to sleep and I would sit and meditate, I would watch them leave their physical bodies and walk through the roof of the house into the night sky to have their nightly adventures. I remember one particular event that was quite spectacular. It was early morning and I was meditating. I suddenly found myself on a spaceship talking to an extraterrestrial woman. In my soul she felt like a long lost friend and I was ecstatic to see her again. She took me through the ship to her room where we sat and talked for a while. In coming out of the meditation, I was surprised at what occurred. I still had no control over my astral experiences, nor did I want to control them. I couldn't remember what we talked about, but I could still remember how the interior of that spaceship looked. All I carried with me was the wonderful feeling of love of having been with her.

I got up after meditating to make breakfast for my son before he went off to school. As soon as he came into the kitchen, he cried,

"Mom, I just had the worst dream! It was so real. There was a spaceship right outside your bedroom window, and I got scared when they took you onboard!"

Many times in talking to people, I can hear their astral bodies talking to me. People tell me one thing and their spirit tells me another. No wonder I was so confused as a child. For example, one day a man came into the store to sell me advertising space in his newspaper. He was very calm and professional, trying to make the sell. His astral body was a totally different matter. It was screaming, "help me, help me, I'm so miserable, I'm going to kill myself." So naturally, I had to say something to him. By this time I had learned how to delicately broach the subject and ask if the person was interested in hearing what I had to say. He told me very bluntly that he wasn't interested, that he didn't want to deal with old issues. A year later he died in a car accident.

On a better note is the story of a young woman who was a customer of the bookstore. We didn't see her for a while, then learned she was suffering from tuberculosis. She was so sick, she had to give up her job, her apartment, and live at home with her parents. She had even broken up with her boyfriend. Months later, she came into the store happy. She had just come from the doctor and learned that her tuberculosis was better, that she didn't need to take medicine anymore.

I heard a totally different story from her spirit, which was telling me that she was getting ready to go out and have a traffic accident because she still didn't want to be better. Fortunately, this woman was more interested in hearing what I had to say.

We talked for an hour and by this time I had fully developed the system. The session was incredible. I am always humbled by the power of the System For Soul Memory. It's like doing five years of therapy in one hour. For the young woman, it was an hour of self-discovery. I got her to feel her emotions. Through where she was feeling them and in what chakra they sat, I was able to pinpoint the age when her problem with tuberculosis first started.

A synopsis of the story goes like this. When she was three, her baby brother was suddenly rushed to the hospital with a severe case of pneumonia. Within a week he was dead. Her parents were never the same afterwards. They were more distant and less loving. Because she was so young, she was not able to understand their change in attitude. She always blamed herself. Not until 23 years later did things make sense. In talking together she saw clearly how she was feeling unloved by her parents. She saw how she had created a lung disease to simulate her brother's ailment, which forced her to live at home so her parents could care for her and love her again. Once she saw all this and cried out all her feelings of despair, powerlessness, and feeling unloved, she left the store feeling like a weight had been lifted from her body. She called three days later to tell me how her life was turning around. She had two new job offers and a date with a guy she had always wanted to go out with.

I hope the System For Soul Memory works for you as it has for me in discovering myself and why I do the things I do. The System will be an important tool in the days to come as the New Age of Enlightenment takes greater hold. Our bodies will need to be free of old blocks so that all the new, faster vibrating energy has the freedom to pass through us and fill us with love and intuitive abilities.

In December of 1995, in a meditation, I experienced the rapture the Bible speaks about as a sign of Armageddon and the coming days of super-consciousness. Since I experience the future in my meditations, I knew then that the days of enlightenment were just around the corner. Paralyzed by the rapture, flooded with such explosive love, was the most incredible feeling I have ever had. It also ended up being the worst. All my old notions of love and God were destroyed. I realized how that much love and energy could not exist on the planet the way we are now. It was too explosive. The earth and its inhabitants were going to have to vibrate faster to accept it. To do that meant that we would have to go through earth changes as well as body changes. In other words, just as we will have to free ourselves of all the old energy blocks in our bodies, the earth too will have to free herself of all the old pollution and negative energy. The journey will be an easy one if we realize that all that is happening is just a shift in energy to accommodate the greater influx of love and God into our lives.

In summing up, I leave you with the one thought that will be the most helpful in the days to come and in using the System For Soul Memory. People who know me are always teasing me because it is the one thing I'm always saying over and over. Remember to "**feel your feelings**." Your emotions are the most important part of you. They are your connection to God. If there is only one thing you learn from this book, I hope this is it.

1

The Energy System of Your Body

Through the years of meditating and being psychic, I've come to understand many things about the energy system of the body. This system is not much different than other systems of the body such as the digestive system, the cardiovascular system, and the nervous system. The energy system also runs quite logically and has specific functions. When I am talking about energy, I am not talking about the electrical system of the body, which uses the brain and the central nervous system. I am talking about an energy system that pulses with subtler, as of yet, unseen subatomic energies. These subatomic energies create a field that surrounds the body. This field is called the aura. The brain has the ability to see and comprehend this energy field. Everyone senses it at one time or another. People, who can instantly size up other people well, are reading this energy field.

This energy field, the aura, can tell you much about a person. It can tell you how a person feels emotionally and physically. Viruses show up in the aura two days before it becomes evident in the body. Not only does the aura show illness, but it also shows when you are getting ready to hurt yourself, or have an accident. Old emotional traumas from the past remain like markers in the aura until they are healed. The energy field shows when a person is lying or telling the truth, when they are feeling passion, thinking and receiving inspiration, feeling happy, angry, and so much more. When I am doing a psychic reading and telling someone their future, I am reading the data from the subatomic particles of that person's energy field.

Science has very little information about this subtle energy system. The Chinese have more information, understanding that there are energy centers in the body called Chakras that work through a series of energy highways called meridians. Acupuncture is based on this. Science would consider this more theory since it does not have the tools to prove this energy exists. But as a psychic, I know this energy exists. I see it surrounding you in your aura. I can hear it, feel it and see the future you are getting ready to attract with it. Why do I see it and you don't? Because I was born with that part of the brain more active. Yet everyone has the ability to know this energy. You can easily be taught to develop this part of the brain and make it more active in your life. This part of the brain does not rely on the five senses—touch, smell, hearing, seeing and tasting, to feed you information about your world. This part of the brain relies on feelings—emotions. Since we are not taught to feel our emotions, this part of the brain rarely gets developed.

In this book I am going to explain about the energy system of your body. I am going to show you how it operates in your life. As a psychic, I have come to learn that the aura is comprised of thoughts and emotions. These thoughts and emotions in conjunction with the soul, are part of an energy system that runs quite logically. Once you understand this system, you will understand yourself— why you think and feel the way you do and why certain things keep happening to you. Understanding this system will help you change your life.

If you stop to consider, most of the time, your thoughts and emotions seem random and out of control. They seem to come from nowhere. Usually they affect your life in minor ways. But sometimes they burst upon you suddenly, with such impact that they dramatically change your life. When this happens, you feel helpless, not having much understanding why this is occurring. How many times have you asked yourself, "Why am I always doing this, why can't I change my attitude, why do I have no control? Why is this happening to me?"

In this book I am going to explain why certain things keep happening to you. Why you think and feel the way you do. I am going to show you how your thoughts and feelings are not arbitrary, but operate quite logically. I am going to show you how they cycle through your energy system in a manor that can be easily explained and changed if desired. I am also going to show you how to feel your emotions. Amazingly, most people don't know how to feel their emotions. They either know how to bury them or to act them out.

Therefore, I ask that you pay attention to how you feel while you are reading this book, especially in the first three chapters when I am asking you to think differently. I am going to take the ten years of meditation, spiritual counseling, and learning about Eastern energy theories I have done, and compile them into a simple, logical approach to give you a new slant about yourself. Once you finish reading this book, you will have a better understanding of yourself. You will know why you do the things you do. You will know how to change the things you want to change.

This system has worked for everyone who has used it. For some, it has changed their lives dramatically. I warn you now; this system is very powerful. If you are not ready to make changes in your life, don't use it! With this system you can no longer be a victim to the circumstances in your life. With this system you will see how you create everything in your life. How you create getting into a car accident, how you get yourself fired from your job, how you make your loved one cheat on you, how you get brain cancer, or make your best friend betray you. Everything!

Does this sound extraordinary to you? Right now you are probably disagreeing with me. Yet I will show you how your life cycles. How you take the energy of your body and continue to recycle it. I will show you how this energy attracts certain events, and how you develop certain patterns in your life.

I will refer to this unseen energy system as the subconscious. Science has made us believe that the subconscious is something hidden, mysterious and very frightening. But it really isn't. We know very little about it, because we don't pay much attention to it. Quite honestly, we pay very little attention to ourselves—to our thoughts and emotions. Most of our attention is focused on the outside world. We are slaves to our five senses. We have been programmed into believing that what we see, touch, smell, taste, and hear is the truth and more important than those 'gut feelings' and anything we may feel or think. After all, we need our five senses for survival.

But I am going to show you that your subconscious is the most important thing in your life. It is your Sixth sense. It creates the circumstances that you later need your five senses for. It is the energy system that runs your body and surrounds you, and it is comprised of your thoughts, emotions, and your soul. Your subconscious creates your future. Once you pay attention to it, you will understand how this happens. Your subconscious won't be so mysterious or scary anymore. Neither will be your feelings.

I want you to begin thinking that there are two parts of yourself: the *Small You* and the *Big You*.

The Small You is the normal you. How you have lived so far. How you have lived *reacting* to life. Think back and notice how most of what you have done is in reaction to something. This reaction is what sets off your five senses.

The Big You is the *creator* you. This is you and the energy field around you— *your subconscious*, your soul, thoughts and emotions. This is the part of you that walks before you, that tunes into things first. It creates your future, senses your surroundings, and the people around you. It is that 'gut feeling'. Your energy field is always sending signals back to you, relaying you information, telling you what to expect. Because you don't have your brain tuned into it, you don't receive those signals.

The System For Soul Memory will teach you how to receive those signals. It is a simple system that when you first look at it you will think to yourself, "This is ridiculous, it is too simple. This won't help me change my life." But it will. The most powerful tools for change are sometimes the simplest ones.

How Your Energy System Works

Physics will tell you that when you look at an object through a highly powered microscope, it will look like an illusion—nothing but space and floating subatomic particles. A solid piece of wood that looks and feels hard, through a microscope will be nothing more but space and dancing subatomic particles—energy. In my meditations, when I entered those higher states of consciousness, I saw everything break down to being pure energy—subatomic particles. Through meditation, I also learned that pure energy has *consciousness*. And what do I mean by consciousness? That energy thinks and *feels*. In other words, that solid piece of wood thinks and feels! I learned that everything is energy, and that all energy thinks and feels. I call this all-encompassing energy, God. Once you know this about energy and truly believe it, you can communicate with that piece of wood. You can communicate with anything. That is the beginning to feeling connected with all life.

In these meditations where I experienced myself as God, the feeling of love was the most overpowering force. In a state of rapture, it is too difficult to think. Because of this, I learned that emotion—love—is the driving force behind everything, even our thoughts. Therefore, through meditation, I learned that everything is energy. All energy is comprised of thoughts and emotions. And that emotion is the force behind everything. In other words, it is the catalyst that triggers the thought and gets energy moving to create the physical experience.

If you look at the word–emotion—and break it down: emotion—**e - motion**, you can easily remember that emotion is *e*nergy in *motion.*

Emotion → Thought → Experience

Emotion - triggers thought - triggers energy moving to create the physical experience

The soul was created to *know* thought and feeling, to record the awareness and the wisdom of it through the physical experience. In every dimension, the physical experience manifests differently. The Beings of Light that I meet in my meditations experience the physical as light. Whenever I have conversations with them, it is done through thought produced holographic images and incredible feelings of love. In our dimension, we know the physical through experiencing it in the physical body through the constraints of time and space, where emotions are polarized, (example: love- hate, sad-happy.)

Your soul computes and remembers everything about you. It computes and remembers every thought and feeling you have had in every dimension. Your soul is like a computer. It stores every detail about all that you have been and will be.

In terms of energy, when you are existing as your pure self, simply as God, your Higher Self, or your Holy Spirit or however you wish to call it, your subatomic particles are vibrating at an incredibly fast frequency. (I am not a student of physics, but by frequency I am referring to the wave action of the sub-atomic particles.) This is what I witnessed in Seventh Dimension, the Golden Realm, where everyone exists as a sun of light. Here, your Spirit vibrates so fast, it can't exist in any other dimension. In terms of emotions, it feels like rapture. And what happens when you are in a state of rapture? Nothing. You are existing in a state of love so paralyzing you don't want to do anything because the love is too wonderful, too incredible, too powerful. When you are in this state, you don't even want to think. Nothing in third dimension can even come close to the love that exists on that other level.

Imagine it this way. You are in Las Vegas, it is night and you are driving down the main strip looking at all the beautiful hotels with their huge glittering neon signs. When you are traveling down the road at five miles per hour, you can look and think about everything: what is printed on the signs, what the people look like walking on the sidewalks. If you speed up a little faster, it gets harder to observe. But let's say you accelerate to 500 miles per hour. At that speed all you can see are glittering lights reflecting off a dark sky. The people, the hotels, and the signs disappear.

So for us to exist in third dimension, the soul must take the power of all that energy and reduce it, slow its vibration, so that we can know the density of this physical plane. It is the job of the soul to act like an energy transformer, to take the energy from your Spirit and slow it down so that you can exist in this dimension, in the physical. This is so you can move, experience, do things, and learn things. As your Spirit, you know you are connected to everything. By the time the soul finishes slowing down your energy, you no longer feel love, or the connection to all things. You feel very alone and separate. It is in this separateness that you will learn your greatest revelations about yourself. Yet it is your desire for the love your soul remembers, and that feeling of being connected again, that propels you through life to find it again.

So one of the jobs of the soul then, is to act like an energy transformer. To control and run the energy of your body. In the physical body, it does this through using a system of energy arteries the Eastern religions call *nadis*. You have thousands of nadis running throughout your body. They are connected to a series of energy centers called *chakras*. Chakra is a Sanskrit word meaning wheel. That is because the energy moves through your chakras like a spinning wheel. You have seven major chakras in your body and hundreds of lesser ones. The nadis carries energy from your soul to each of these energy centers, then transfer the energy from the chakras to the rest of your body, through more energy pathways called meridians. Each chakra has a specific function in how it uses and stores the energy. In the following chapters I will explain the specific functions of each chakra.

The soul actually has shape and as of yet can only be seen by the psychic eye. (Once science has mastered the viewing of subatomic particles, the soul will be seen.) The soul is pyramid shaped. It resides as a very bright golden-white light in the chest, with its apex resting at the bottom of the throat and its base against the diaphragm. Have you ever felt so much love that you have felt it tug or pull against your gut? If you have, then you have experienced the soul expanding. 'Gut feelings' is your soul talking to you. If you continue to pay attention to this part of your body, you will discover how your emotions make the soul expand and contract. You will begin to feel the soul as a muscle.

So one of the jobs of the soul is to act like an energy transformer, to take the incredible energy of your spirit and defuse it so you can exist in a body. This energy then continues to cycle through the body, through the energy arteries and centers of your body. As the energy moves, it encounters resistance, which slows the energy even further. This resistance comes in the form of your cells, and within your cells, your DNA. Your DNA is the emotional, mental and physical condition that you have inherited. It is also the lessons you have come into this life to learn. The more energy slows, the denser, more physical it becomes. Once it interacts with your cells, it slows enough to be picked up by the glands and the central nervous system, where it is then relayed to the body in a more physical, electrical manner. What you resist in learning will slow the energy even further, creating energy blocks. Blocked energy leads to illness or physical catastrophe. Too much blocked energy will eventually lead to death.

Science believes that the central nervous system runs the body, relaying messages from the brain and the glands. Yet in reality, the body has already been sent the information through the subatomic energy of the soul. Think of a cell. Every cell has a nucleus that powers it. Only now science is realizing that within the nucleus is an even greater power source of even more finite particles. This is the source I am talking about. These particles comprise the energy field that make up the soul.

Quantum physics is just beginning to discover that subatomic particles can speak to each other across wide distances outside the speed of light. This phenomenon is called 'quantum entanglement.'[1] Through meditation and my psychic experiences, I have learned that *all* subatomic particles speak to each other. To me, it is God recognizing Himself and speaking to Himself. Remember, all energy has consciousness.

Now imagine once again, the soul as a computer. It has an energy source, transforming the incredible power of your Spirit. It also has memory, storing all that you have been and ever will be. But most important, your soul has a programming chip. This chip has been programmed by your Spirit and directs everything about you. What you will learn in this life, what you will look like, what you will do, how you will act, feel, etc.

In the physical body, your programming chip will be your DNA. It will store every detail about all the lifetimes and experiences of your ancestors that will coincide and match the programming chip in your soul. They are both connected. All that exists within your soul exists within your genes. As the saying goes: 'as above, so below.' Whatever is found in spirit will also be found in the physical. Therefore, your DNA has been predisposed by what exists in your soul. You can't have one without the other. They are both one and the same.

Your purpose for being here in third dimension is quite simply to know your DNA. When you learn your DNA, why you are the way you are, why you think and feel the way you do, you will be learning what is in your soul, and what God has planned for you.

The System For Soul Memory is a system I have created that will help you learn this. It will help you understand the energy of your body and what it tells you. Remember, on its most basic level, everything is energy. And all energy has consciousness—thoughts and emotions. On your most basic level, you are the energy of your thoughts and emotions. Your life is a reflection of what you think and feel.

And why would you want to know what this energy tells you?

You wouldn't, not if everything in your life was running smoothly. But what happens when you get sick, or are constantly unhappy? Or if there is something in your life that's not working right and you wish to change it? That is a sign that your energy system is blocked somewhere. That is a sign that you are resisting learning one of your lessons, what you have come here to know.

When your energy system is blocked, the soul will do whatever it must to clear the block. How does it do this? By creating even greater difficulties for you until you finally 'get' what it is trying to tell you. Right now reading this, you are probably in a panic wondering how to go about 'getting' what the soul is trying to tell you. That's because you've been there, watching something in your life go from bad to worse. You know what it's like to be on a downward spiral where one bad thing after another happens, and you don't know how to stop it. We've all been there.

Don't worry the System For Soul Memory will show you how to get out of those ruts. It will help you make your life easier, by helping you to understand yourself better and why you do the things you do. Once you know this, you will be able to work with your soul, the computer you, and change the things that no longer serve you and create the things you want.

2

The Premise of the System

For you to understand the System For Soul Memory, it will be important for you to understand the structure in which the system is founded. This system is based on several conclusions I have made through years of observation and meditation. These conclusions came in different ways.

My first introduction to the chakras came from Swami Paramananda Saraswatti, the channeler for Mafu, when I was studying with the Mastery Program at the Foundation For Meditative Studies in Eagle Point, Oregon. Mafu's presentation of the chakras is unique in that he looks at the chakras through the symbol of the yin/yang.[2] Therefore, the colors ascribed to each chakra are different than what most people teach. In the market place, there are many different books and opinions written about the chakras and their colors. They are all valid. For every level of consciousness or awareness, there is a truth. That is why there are so many religions and belief systems in the world. All roads lead to the same destination, to God. The chakric system you attract, will be the one you require at that particular time of your life, and at your particular level of consciousness. I attracted Mafu's version, which led me into creating this system.

Another way I received information about the chakras came through my meditations. Information would pour through me and I would write it down. In the days and weeks that followed, people and events would come into my life to show me how this information worked. I would have a mental, emotional and a physical 'knowing' of the information for myself. I then saw the profound effect it had on others.

The third way I received information was through spiritual counseling sessions for others. While doing a session, many times I would psychically hear specific questions to ask the client. I discovered these questions always had a purpose. This purpose was to release an old buried hurt, or in other words, blocked energy in a chakra. As emotions surfaced, I was then told to observe the client's reactions. I was also told to observe my own reactions, since many times because of my psychic ability, I would feel their emotion before they did. I began learning more about the chakras this way. I learned how energy feels, and where emotions sit. Sometimes a client's aura became visible so that I could see how the emotion appeared in their energy field. If the client wanted to deal with the emotion, then I would have a psychic vision of the seed pattern, of how that energy originally became blocked. These visions always precipitated the client to be healed.

Patterns began emerging. Slowly I learned how to communicate what I felt and saw. Getting people to understand was the hardest part. Taking a concept that I knew as a feeling and applying it in mundane terms was a challenge. In the beginning, when I talked about the importance of emotions, people looked at me as though I was speaking a foreign language. With some people, it took years for them to understand the concept. This forced me to learn an easier method to get them to know and feel their emotions. I saw the simple, yet difficult steps people needed to heal themselves and change their lives. All of this information grew slowly into a system. It was while I was meditating that the name came to me: The System For Soul Memory; for it is what the soul remembers that makes us look the way we do, act the way we do, and have the life we live. The following premises are the basis for this system.

Premise 1

"Behold, the man is become as one of us, to know good and evil;" (Genesis 3:22). Spoken by God after Adam and Eve ate from the Tree of Knowledge.

Earth is a school, an adventure. We come here to learn, to experience, to gain wisdom, and to know. As I stated previously, when we are in spirit, in 'paradise,' we cannot know good and evil. In paradise, we exist as pure light, in a state of rapture where love is the overwhelming commodity. In order to learn and gain wisdom we must leave paradise and enter a dimension where the energies are slower, denser; where everything appears separate; where even the emotion, love, appears separate, and looks and feels like different emotions. Third dimensional Earth is such a place.

In third dimension we have the necessary ingredients to act out and feel our experiences. We have time: the rising and setting of the sun, day and night, the changing of the seasons which gives us the feeling of past, present and future. We have the six directions: North, South, East, and West, and up and down, which give us the feeling of space, of movement, that we are going somewhere. And we have polarity: yin/yang, opposites, 'good and evil' to learn what we want and don't want.

Love is an easy emotion to feel. It is our natural state of being. But the separate, opposite emotions of love, like hate, betrayal, and abandonment, are much harder to feel because they go against our natural condition. That is why we are here. To learn what we are not.

In premise 1, The System For Soul Memory believes that there is only one way to learn a lesson, and that is through transcendence. Transcendence is a term often applied to meditating. It is a high state of meditation where according to Eastern thought, man goes outside the realm of third dimension and experiences himself as God through his Spirit. The more a person meditates and experiences transcendence, the more God-like the person becomes.

In my experiences of meditating, I discovered transcendence to be a state of total awareness. This is a condition where I am in a state of *high emotion*, where every thought and every physical movement is intensely experienced. Have you ever listened to music that was so moving and absorbing that you began to cry? At that moment you were in a state of transcendence. In doing counseling sessions with clients, I discovered that this same requirement must be achieved in order for a lesson to be learned. Transcendence must be experienced. You must be in a state of high emotion where the thought and physical condition of the experience must be keenly felt and observed.

For the soul to gain wisdom, it must have awareness through body, mind and soul. Body represents the actual physical experience. Mind represents the thought or conscious awareness of the experience. And soul represents the emotional or subconscious/ unconscious awareness.

Many times a client will come to me with a reoccurring pattern in their life they wish to change. Some of these people have been in therapy working on the issue. Yet, even with therapy, they have not been able to work through the issue and make the necessary changes in their life. In talking to these people I discovered that many times they have a mental awareness of their problem, but not the intense, emotional awareness. They may be able to tell me the emotion they are feeling, but many times they have not actually felt the emotion fully. That is why their pattern is still continuing. Until they fully feel the emotion, and fulfill the requirements of transcendence, they will not be able to make the necessary changes in their life. In Chapter 13, I explain how to feel an emotion.

Therefore, Premise 1 of the System For Soul Memory is that Earth is a school of learning and that we come to Earth to gain wisdom. The only way the soul can gain wisdom is through transcendence: through the physical, mental and emotional awareness of an experience.

Premise 2

The System For Soul Memory believes that the language of the soul is emotion. In order to speak to the soul, you must speak to it in the language it knows. If you have ever had a spiritual experience, you will know what I am talking about. All spiritual experiences are flooded with love. God speaks to us through the emotion of love. To us in Third Dimension where polarity operates and everything is separate, love breaks down to being every emotion: love, hate, happy, sad, betrayal, trust, abandonment, etc. So when our souls get programmed, they are programmed in the language of emotion. As I stated previously, emotion is the underlying propellant that triggers our thoughts and actions. It is the way energy operates. Every action we take has an emotion lying behind it, causing it to happen. Most of the time we go through life not aware of our emotions. Even the simple act of going to work, playing football, going to the grocery store, interacting with people, all have underlying emotions. If you think about it, you will be able to figure out what they are. They will be different for each person based on the uniqueness of each life.

Knowing that emotion is the language of the soul is a shortcut to making changes in your life. Just feeling the emotion of a situation will automatically trigger the mental and physical awareness. By feeling the emotion, you are talking directly to God and to your soul. You are making changes without going through the long process of having the soul create an incident to get you to react, to feel the emotion. You only need to know the emotion causing the situation to begin making changes in your life. The mental and physical aspects will automatically come later. Emotional awareness, mental awareness and physical awareness do not have to occur simultaneously for a lesson to be learned.

Therefore, Premise 2 of the System For Soul Memory believes that the language of the soul is emotion. To speak to the soul, to make changes in your life, you must use emotion. Emotion is what triggers our thoughts and actions. Each experience we have has an emotion underlying it.

Premise 3

How do you know what your learning lessons are? The System For Soul Memory believes that your DNA, your genetic makeup is your learning lesson. *You are here simply to know yourself.* Your soul carries with it memories from all that you have been in all dimensions throughout eternity. Your family on earth has been specially selected to coincide with what is in your soul; what you hope to learn and what you wish to accomplish. Just look at your parents and your ancestors. Besides having inherited their physical makeup, you have also inherited their mental and emotional makeup. What your parents didn't learn, you will be learning. In other words, the emotions they didn't process will be the same emotions you will be processing. That is why you see inherited tendencies, such as addiction and abuse, running through families generation after generation. The emotions behind these tendencies are difficult to process.

There will also be goals and desires you hope to accomplish in your life. These tendencies are fired by emotions that are also inherited. If you are an artist, musician, writer, builder, teacher, look back at your ancestors and you will find someone in the family with the same desires. You may be acting out the tendency a little differently. For instance, no one in my family meditated, but my grandmother did spend every morning praying. The emotion behind both actions is the same.

Also, the emotions and desires from one generation to the next may go one step further in the next generation. I call this the **snowball effect.** If you ever watched the Olympics, you saw how old records were constantly being broken. In each progressive generation, people are running faster, jumping higher, and demonstrating more skill.

This can also be seen on a more negative note. Disease can show up in a family where it never existed before. The System For Soul Memory believes that an emotion that is not dealt with progressively from one generation to the next can get so deeply buried, it can change the genetic makeup of the family.

Genetic makeup is always mutating.[3] The System For Soul Memory believes that when you gain the wisdom of an experience, you change your genetic makeup. Disease is one of the last attempts the soul makes to get you to feel an emotion. A buried emotion is the reason that disease occurs in the first place. In any disease, permanent healing can only happen when the buried emotion has been fully felt and realized on a conscious level. Transcendence must be fulfilled. When the gene has been changed, it has been changed for future generations. Watch what happens to your parents and your children once you have learned something. Your changing changes them.

Premise 3 of the System For Soul Memory states that your learning lessons are written in your DNA. What you have inherited is what you are here to learn.

Premise 4

The System For Soul Memory believes that the energy of your body develops chakra by chakra through the first eight years of your life. In other words, the energy field grows and develops slowly just as the physical body does. Beginning with the Root Chakra, each chakra takes roughly one year to develop. The only exception is the Root Chakra, which begins developing at the moment of conception and continues through the first year of life. Besides the 7 major chakras, the System For Soul Memory also includes the Moon Center Chakra in the development of the

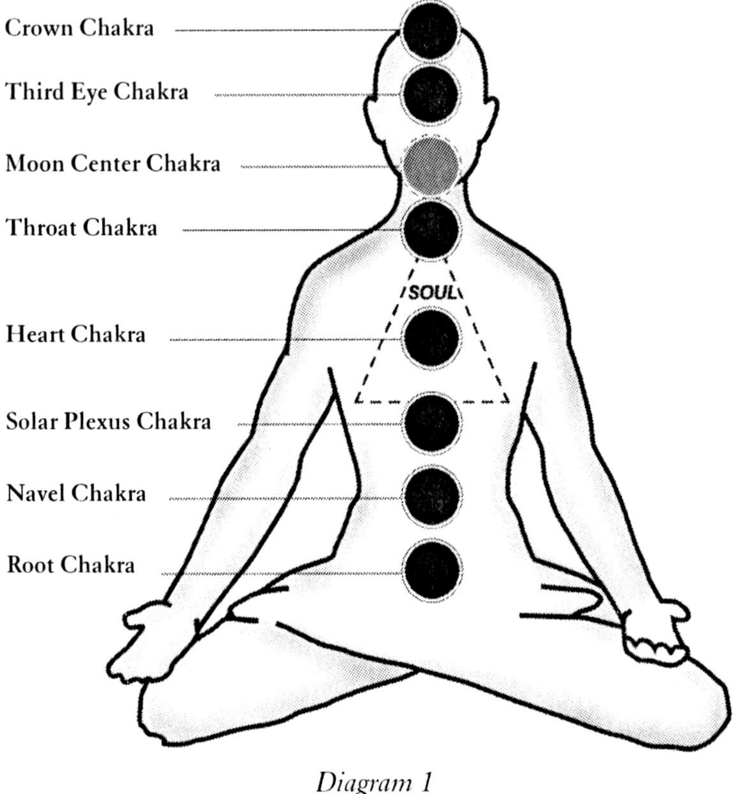

Diagram 1

body's energy system. The Moon Center Chakra is found at the back of the neck at the top of the spine. (See Diagram 1) In Eastern studies, this chakra is generally associated with the Third Eye Chakra since they are connected. In working with people, I found the Moon Center Chakra to be one of the most important in soul growth. This is why it is included in the System For Soul Memory.

Throughout the year that each chakra develops, the soul presents for the first time the lessons you are here to learn. Each lesson is presented as an emotion, since that is the language of the soul. These emotions then trigger the physical events in your life to occur.

The System For Soul Memory believes that each chakra has a particular set of emotions that resonate to it. Therefore, this creates a similar grouping of emotions to exist in each chakra. This grouping creates a developmental theme. For example, all the emotions found in the Heart Chakra deal with love and affect our relationships.

As I have stated, each emotion in each chakra triggers a physical event to occur. These events occur during the year that chakra is developing. For example, let us take the Heart Chakra again. It develops at the age of four. Its theme of development deals with love and relationships. If abandonment is one of the lessons to be learned, then at the age of four an event will occur to make the person aware he is being abandoned. In Chapters 5-12 you can read in detail about each of the chakras.

On the physical level, your DNA has been programmed with this roadmap for your development. This roadmap contains all the emotions you will experience throughout your life, and has been programmed by the soul to coincide with the development of the chakras through the first eight years. By the time you are nine years old, you will have experienced every emotion you are here to learn.

Once again, you will experience these emotions, your learning lessons, through the normal events of your life. Look at your life up until this point; think about all your experiences, your likes and dislikes, your patterns, and you will see which emotions are stored in your soul. You will see what you are here to learn.

The *emotions* not felt during the first eight years of life will be stored in the chakras as *energy*. Throughout your life, the soul continues to recycle the emotion until you feel it. The soul does this by creating physical events to get you to react to a situation. In reacting to a situation, the emotion that was previously buried is brought to the surface allowing you the ability to feel it once again.

Therefore, Premise 4 states that the soul will present your learning lessons to you through the first eight years of your life through the development of each Chakra. This will manifest as specific emotions for each chakra. Every emotion you will ever know will be presented at this time. They will be stored in the chakras until you learn them, and will trigger the events of your life.

Premise 5

There are only two ways the energy of an emotion can be released once it is stored in the chakra. The first way is the simplest way, and that is by feeling the emotion. By having transcendent awareness of it. In this way the emotion is released as energy.

The second way seems to be the more common way. In this way, emotions are constantly repressed, until the energy in the chakra gets so dense it becomes physical matter. This matter will show up as a physical malady in the body, such as disease, cancer, broken bones, burns, cuts, scrapes, muscle tears, etc. The severity of the injury or illness will tell you how repressed the emotion is and how dense the energy has become. Therefore, the second way the energy of an emotion gets released is through physical matter.

Once emotion is trapped in physical matter, there are two ways to heal. Either, the diseased or injured part of the body is removed; or the trapped emotion is felt and released as energy. You can read more about this in Chapter 16.

The soul wants you to feel the emotion as energy. Therefore, even after the emotion has turned to physical matter, the soul continues to create events to get you to experience and feel the emotion that is trapped. It does this throughout the healing process.

The way an injury or illness occurs is important. How you get hurt helps you feel and release blocked emotions. For example, when Roger was growing up he felt powerless to his father. Recently he began working for a man who reminded him of his father. Every time he had to be with him, he felt the same sense of helplessness. Instead of feeling the helplessness, Roger tried to think up ways of getting around it. Roger repressed the emotion to the point where he created a car accident. In the accident, Roger was hit by a man who ran a red light. His car was totaled and he was trapped in the front seat. The feeling of helplessness overwhelmed him as he waited for the 'jaws of life' to come and free him. Roger suffered broken bones in his right leg. His recovery period once again created the feeling of helplessness. He couldn't get around easily; therefore, he missed several weeks of work. How fully Roger feels the emotion during this time will determine how quickly the injury heals. If the injury never fully heals, then the emotion was not fully felt.

If an emotion is even more repressed and the physical trauma is more severe like cancer or disease, emotion will be released through the highs and lows of the healing process. Creating a life-threatening situation is the last resort for the soul. If healing does not take place, and the emotion is not felt, death will follow. Energy in the body will be so badly blocked, there won't be enough life force to sustain it. By this time, the soul has done all that it can to get you to feel the emotion.

For example, Walter doesn't feel right. He's got a cold that won't go away. He visits his doctor who takes x-rays and doesn't find anything wrong. Walter is given antibiotics and told to return in a couple of weeks if the problem persists. Five months and three doctors later, Walter discovers he has lung cancer. By this time the cancer is also found in tissue surrounding his heart, making the cancer inoperable. The only thing that may help Walter is a new, expensive, experimental drug his HMO won't pay for. Walter feels betrayed.

Using the System For Soul Memory, Walter tries to remember the first eight years of his life, but can't. He does remember though, feeling betrayed in high school, when he was failing geometry. He asked his parents for help, but they were too overwhelmed with work, and with caring for his other brothers and sisters to help him. Walter then asked his math teacher to stay after school and help him. But his teacher was coaching soccer league, and couldn't help either. So the teacher recommended that Walter hire a tutor. His family could not afford it. No one helped Walter. He ended up flunking the class and taking it again in summer school. The emotions he buried as a teenager, betrayal, helplessness and humiliation, are the same emotions Walter re-experienced during his health crisis.

Premise 5 of the System For Soul Memory gives you two ways to release the energy of an emotion. The first way is by simply feeling it. The second way is through injury or illness, through physical matter.

Premise 6

The first time a learning lesson is presented during the first eight years of life, an energy pattern is established. The System For Soul Memory believes that *how* an emotion first gets introduced is very important in how that emotion gets recycled later through life. The events surrounding the introduction of the emotion create an energy pattern of certain behavioral and thought patterns. Everything in your environment will be part of this pattern. This includes where you were, what you were doing, what you were wearing, eating and even thinking. This energy pattern will be the basis for future events when the emotion next gets triggered. This pattern will cause you to act out your emotion in a specific way. The System For Soul Memory calls this a **seed pattern**.

For instance, Rosemary was raised by a mother who was physically abusive. The first time her mother viciously struck her was at the Thanksgiving dinner table when she was four years old. The emotion Rosemary experienced was abandonment. Later in life, whenever Rosemary felt abandoned, she would act out her anger at the dinner table. The dinner table was the scene where her first experience with abandonment occurred, and it was the place where she felt most vulnerable. Later in her life, the dinner table was the place where she told her husband she wanted a divorce. The dinner table was the place when the urge to strike her children was the strongest. These actions were all done subconsciously. Rosemary had no conscious awareness of why the urge to strike her children came at this particular time or place. Curiously, Rosemary also had an allergy to turkey.

Or take the case of Henry. When Henry was seven, his parents took a trip to Europe for six weeks, leaving Henry alone for the first time with a babysitter. While his parents were away, Henry had an accident. He fell off his bike and badly bumped his head. Not having his parents at home to console him made Henry feel sad. Later in life, while Henry was getting a divorce, he suffered from debilitating headaches. It wasn't until we talked that Henry realized how his subconscious had associated bumping his head and headaches, with the feeling of abandonment. Instead of feeling the emotion of abandonment, Henry acted it out by reliving his seed pattern.

Another example would be the case of Jean. When she was six years old, her father took her to the toy store in the mall to spend the Christmas money she just received. As they approached the check out line, Jean could not find the money. Her father made a big scene in the store, in front of the long line of people waiting to check out, and called Jean stupid for losing her money. When Jean became an adult she loved going shopping in malls. So much so that she became deeply in debt owing the credit card companies thousands of dollars. When I asked Jean what she felt when she thought about owing so much money, she replied that she felt stupid. After helping her feel the emotion, it was easy for Jean to see the connection between her money problems and the incident when she was six. In her subconscious, Jean associated malls as being a place where she felt stupid. Jean acted out the emotion by overspending, proving over and over that she was stupid. Jean's overspending stopped as soon as she realized her seed pattern, and felt all the emotions involved.

The System For Soul Memory believes that the easiest way to learn a lesson and have transcendent awareness of an emotion is by remembering the seed pattern, when the emotion was first introduced. Many times I witnessed how much easier it was for a client to remember a particular incident that occurred during the first eight years of their lives, and to feel their pain as a child. As soon as they did, an instantaneous knowing occurred. They immediately saw how that incident created a pattern in their life. Having this knowing changed their life instantly. How? By having conscious awareness of it. If the pattern emerged again, they immediately recognized it. There was no longer an issue with it.

When you fully feel the emotion, you will no longer experience the situation again. You will know you learned your lesson when the pattern leaves your life. That particular emotion will no longer be a problem. In the future, you may feel it again, but it will be easily felt. Your thoughts will be different, too. You will have more compassion for those who have suffered the same. You will be able to forgive those that hurt you. You may even notice a change physically. You will have changed the energy pattern of your body.

Premise 6 states that an energy pattern is established the first time a lesson is presented. This energy pattern causes you to act and think in a particular way every time the emotion re-emerges. This is called a seed pattern. The seed pattern is established in the first eight years of life and will be the subconscious basis for future experiences.

Premise 7

Like energy attracts like energy. Throughout your life you will attract people with similar energy to yours. What is meant by similar energy? People with the same learning lessons. The soul is a magnet. It will attract the necessary people and events into your life until you 'know' what you are here to learn. Each person who comes into your life is a mirror of you, reflecting one of the emotions you are here to learn. These people are going to help you learn your lesson as you are going to help them learn theirs. It is by mutual consent on a subconscious level that you are in each other's life.

It is the job of the soul to make sure you learn your lessons. The soul will continue to recycle your emotions, until you know them. The soul uses the **snowball effect** to get you to feel your emotions. In the beginning of the recycling process, the soul presents the lesson as gently as a 'snowflake.' In other words, it is presented as a minor daily occurrence. Someone may say something in passing that will offend you, or cut you off while driving, or take credit for something you did at work, etc., etc. All of these actions are intended by the soul to get you to react, to feel the emotion underlying the action.

If you don't feel the emotion at this time, the soul then takes this 'snowflake' incident and begins to *snowball* it, or enlarge it. In other words the next time the soul reintroduces the emotion, it may trigger a major fight with someone, instead of the previous, minor insult. You may get into a car accident with someone, instead of just being cut off. Or you may be bypassed for a promotion, instead of not being recognized. If you continue to be hardhearted and not feel the emotion, the soul will continue *snowballing* the incident until it becomes an avalanche in your life. This avalanche will occur as a life-changing situation, like a divorce, or a major injury or illness, or a loss of job and security. The soul will do what it must to get you to notice. It will stop your life, put you into shock, and shake you up until you can do nothing but look at the emotion and feel it. Does this sound familiar? I always recommend to clients to feel their emotions while they are still snowflakes. Life is so much easier that way. Unfortunately, most clients come to me after the avalanche has hit.

When you begin to use the System For Soul Memory you will be able to avoid the avalanches in your life. You will train yourself to attune to your emotions and feel them while they are still snowflakes. That is how the System For Soul Memory makes your life easier.

In Premise 7, the System For Soul Memory believes that the soul will attract to you those individuals with similar learning lessons, to create the events necessary for you to learn your lesson. The soul will continue to recycle your lesson, creating more drastic events each time the lesson gets presented, until you finally know it.

Premise 8

For every action, there is an equal reaction. This applies to emotions, too. Polarity is basic when discussing emotional energy. When learning an emotion, you will be learning both sides of the emotion. For example, you will be learning good/ bad, love/hate, pride/humility, generosity/greediness, happy/sad, etc. Referring once again to the Bible and Genesis, God told Adam he would be learning both 'good and evil.' In other words, once the energy of good has been created, at the same time, the energy of evil takes form. Once you realize that you will be dealing with the polarities of an emotion, that they will both come and go in your life, you will be better prepared to deal with them.

It is easy to feel the good emotions. It is difficult to feel the bad ones. Those are the ones we tend to bury and go out of our way not to feel. In this book, I will mainly write about the difficult emotions.

I always tell people to think about a pendulum. A pendulum is balanced by swinging both ways equally. The same applies to humans. In order to be in balance, you must allow both sides of an emotion to emerge and be felt equally. This is what creates contentment and peace in life.

When you try to control the swing of the pendulum, you go out of balance. Every time you *think* of a way to avoid feeling an emotion, you are trying to control the swing of the pendulum. Let's take the issue of feeling like a success or failure. To be in balance you must realize that at certain times in your life you will feel like a success and at other times you will feel like a failure. Let's take John as an example.

John grew up with a gambler for a father. His father's addiction was always causing havoc at home during John's early years. Several times John would have to move due to the financial difficulties created by his father. When John was seventeen his parents finally got divorced. By this time John hated his father and vowed never to be like him. He never wanted to speak to him again.

John polarized his father's addiction. Intent on not being a failure, John became a workaholic. He started out as an electrician, and worked very hard, building a large, electrical contracting company. This came at a price, though. John worked so hard, he didn't get to spend much time with his wife and two children. Then suddenly, things began to change. A recession hit, and new construction fizzled. John's sales began to slide. John took money out of his own pocket to pay his employees when times got particularly slow. He tried many new approaches to increase sales, even calling in the experts, but nothing seemed to work. He was losing his business.

The stress during this period changed John. His wife didn't like it and began to complain. It was bad enough that she had been ignored all those years while he was too busy working. But now he had become even more remote, burying himself in his own problems. His wife threatened to divorce him.

At first John didn't see that he was just like his father, living out his father's life. After all he had spent most of his life proving he was different. But the genes don't lie. The circumstances may have been different, but the underlying issue was the same. In both cases the soul wanted to know what it felt like to be a failure. In both cases, the obsession, in the father's case, gambling, and in the son' case, overworking, allowed each man to act out the emotion instead of feel it. In both cases the end result was still the same: failure.

At first when John realized this, he was very angry. He felt his whole life was for nothing. He was terrified of feeling the emotion of failure. He associated it with abandonment and being alone. That's what happened to his father when his wife and children left him. Now it was happening to John. John kept ignoring the 'snowflakes' his soul was putting into his life. Now his soul was creating an 'avalanche'. John had no choice but to recognize and feel his emotions

It took John a while to get through to his emotions, and to learn how to feel them. Every time the feeling of being a failure came up, John's natural inclination was to act it out by working harder. It was difficult for him to learn to sit still and feel the emotion. But once he did, he didn't care anymore whether his business turned around or not; he cared more about his wife and family. Feeling his own failure helped him to understand himself better. This in turn helped him understand his father better. John could now let the past go. He was able to forgive his father.

Almost immediately, John noticed an improvement in business. His soul no longer required him to be a failure; therefore, John no longer acted like a failure. People noticed the change in him. John learned his lesson and his energy system changed. Six months later, after his business began showing a profit again, John received a telephone call from his father. Healing had occurred, wisdom was gained, and the soul was presenting John with the final chapter to learning his lesson: making peace with his father.

Premise 8 states that when learning an emotion, you will be learning both sides of the emotion, its polarity.

3

How the System for Soul Memory Works

For the last ten years I have been learning about the soul, the energy system of the body and our emotions. This process is still ongoing and I still find it humbling and fascinating. What you are about to read is what I learned so far. It has taken me many years to simplify this information. In the beginning, this information challenged some of my previously held beliefs. These beliefs were based on what I read previously concerning chakras and auras. What I know now makes more sense. It takes the concept of the 'soul' and applies it in a more mundane fashion. No longer is the soul an imaginary spiritual concept, but an actual physical presence that, with practice, can be felt and understood. I have taken the information I learned and condensed it into a system I call the System For Soul Memory. This system tells of the soul's purpose, how it operates in our life, how it operates in conjunction with the energy system of our body, and how we can use this system to tap into our soul to change the quality of our life. Once again I will reiterate what I have written.

How the Soul Gains Wisdom

As I stated previously, we come to earth to learn, to know. There is only one way the soul can learn, and that is through transcendence: the knowing of an experience through mental, emotional and physical awareness.

Emotion is the language of God. Our souls are programmed with the emotions we are here to learn. And how do we learn them? We learn them by acting them out and thinking about them. In other words, these emotions are our *subconscious*. They trigger our thoughts and create the physical events in our life to happen. It is through our *reaction* to these physical events that we then have *conscious* awareness of what these emotions are. To simplify:

1. God programs our soul with the emotions we are here to learn.
2. These emotions then create the physical events in our daily life.
3. Each event causes us to react. This reaction illuminates what is subconscious, and makes it conscious.
4. When an event occurs, in order to gain wisdom from it, we must be aware of:
   a. the *physical* circumstances surrounding the event,
   b. our *thoughts* concerning the event,
   c. but most especially, the *emotions* we felt during the event
5. If this criteria is not met, if there is not conscious awareness to all three, then the soul stores the emotion in the chakras, and replays it in the future through the creation of another event.

The soul creates a specific event to get you to feel a specific emotion. If you don't *feel* the emotion, then the soul guarantees you will *live* the emotion until you do. In other words, the soul will continue to create more of the same events until you do finally feel it.

The Energy System of Your Body

The soul uses the energy system of your body to present your learning lessons to you. According to the System For Soul Memory, this energy system is comprised of 8 main energy centers called chakras. Within the chakras are energy arteries or passageways called *nadis*. These nadis connect the chakras to each other, then branch out further to connect each chakra to the glands and organs of the body. From the glands and organs run more energy highways called *meridians* which branch out to the rest of the body. You can picture it like the central nervous system of your body, with nerves branching out from the spinal column to the rest of your body; or like the circulatory system with veins and arteries running from the heart to every part of your body. This entire energy system encompasses and surrounds your body. It radiates anywhere from several inches beyond your body to many miles, depending on how spiritual you are, or on how you use your energy. The average radius is a couple of feet, yet I found people who perform before large audiences to unconsciously train their auras to extend much farther.

The energy system of your body is managed by the soul. This whole system is subatomic and is constantly receiving information from everything, everywhere. It receives information from the environment, from animals, from the people around you, from your spirit, and the spirit world. The soul takes this information and sends it to your chakras. It begins by passing this information out your back, between your shoulder blades. (Remember, your soul sits in your chest, behind your heart, between your diaphragm and your throat. I found this area of the back to be extremely sensitive and receptive to the energies of others and think of it as the 'eyes' in back of my head.) From your back, the information then travels up, behind your neck, over your head, down through the Crown Chakra, then down through the *shushumna*, the main nadis-passageway found in the spine, to the rest of your chakras and their connecting nadis. Each chakra spins clockwise, the nadis in each chakra striving to synchronize in unison with the nadis of the other chakras to create a perfect balance of spinning chakras. I say striving. Blocked emotions are what prevent the chakras from spinning uniformly.

At this level, the subatomic energy feels emotional. Each emotion vibrates to its own frequency, just as each chakra vibrates to its own frequency. Therefore, the frequency of certain emotions resonate to a particular chakra. As the energy passes down through the Crown Chakra to the other chakras, the frequency of the chakra determines where the information sent by the soul resides. This frequency also creates the color of each chakra and the colors found in your aura. Once this information settles into a chakra, it is then picked up by the gland of that chakra. The gland, through the hormones and the electrical frequencies of the central nervous system, then relays the information to the brain, the organs, and the rest of the body. You will know this information as your thoughts and emotions, and the impulses you have to act them out.

How the Energy System Develops

Your energy system develops through the first eight years of your life through the unfolding process of each chakra. Beginning with the Root Chakra and ending with the Crown Chakra, each chakra takes roughly one year to unfold. I say roughly because each individual is unique in its development. Just as some people reach puberty at an early age, some will develop their chakras a little faster or a little slower depending on the personality of the spirit and the corresponding DNA in the body. Also, don't forget that the Root Chakra begins developing at the time of conception and continues through the first year of life.

It is during each chakra's year of development that the soul presents for the first time, those emotions you are here to learn and know. Each chakra carries a theme of development and harbors those emotions that resonate to that theme.

In the unfolding process, the way the emotion is first presented establishes an energy pattern that gets recycled throughout the rest of your life until the emotion is learned. This pattern is called a *seed pattern*. What this means is that every time after the first eight years when the emotion next surfaces, attached to the emotion is a memory of how that emotion was first experienced. This memory creates a specific pattern of thought and behavior so that the next time the emotion arises, you will act and think the same you way did the first time, even though the circumstances will be different.

The Recycling Process

After the first eight years, the soul begins to recycle whatever emotions are still stored in the chakras. These will be the emotions not originally felt. The soul reintroduces them into your life to get you to deal with them. The soul continues this recycling process until you learn all your lessons.

When the soul reintroduces an emotion, you have seven years to feel the emotion and release it. If you don't, then the **snowball effect** goes into action. In other words, if you do not work through an emotion through the seven-year cycle, then for the next cycle, when the soul reintroduces the emotion again, the circumstances will be harsher and more traumatic.

I find that most people are working on more than one chakra at a time. Most diseases are a combination of severely blocked emotions coming from different chakras. Also, one event can have several emotions triggering it. Remember the story about work-aholic John and his gambling father. Even though John was working on the issue of success and failure, he also had the emotion of abandonment attached to it. Once John finished working through his feeling of failure, the next step the soul presented to him was that phone call from his father. Talking to his father brought up the old buried feeling of abandonment. On an energy level, these emotions are found in different chakras. It is the nadis that connect them together.

There are also other triggers that cause the soul to release a buried emotion and create an incident. One such trigger will be your children. The development of their chakras in the first eight years of their life can trigger the release of the same emotion in you, especially if that emotion was inherited.

Take for example the case of Jim. When Jim was a baby, his family moved into a new house. Because his mother spent more time unpacking and getting settled than watching after him, Jim didn't feel safe in his new surroundings. He developed a severe case of psoriasis. It wasn't until Jim got married and his wife got pregnant, that the psoriasis appeared again. Knowing that the baby was coming, Jim had a strong urge to move, even though the house they lived in was adequate to accommodate the three of them. Jim just didn't feel comfortable. It wasn't until we spoke that he realized the connection. The development of the Root Chakra in that of his child triggered the emotions of safety blocked in his own Root Chakra.

The traumas of friends and loved ones can also trigger a similar emotion in you. Remember, like energy attracts like energy. You and your friends will be working on similar issues. Also, anything physical that makes your five senses react, like a special food, a smell, or a song, etc. can also trigger a long ago hurt.

The trauma of a pet can also have a strong impact on triggering a buried hurt. Working as an animal psychic, I witnessed over and over how the problem of a pet will mirror a problem of the owner. Take for example the case of Chula the Cat. Chula lived in an apartment in New York City. For no apparent reason, one day, Chula refused to use her litter box. She began urinating all over the apartment. Mr. and Mrs. Fields, the couple who owned her, were frantic. They could not understand the sudden change in the cat. When I spoke to Chula, the cat relayed through mental images and emotions, the story. She told me she was feeling very lonely. The owners were working longer hours and traveling more, and they were ignoring her. Chula felt abandoned. Chula also told me that she had met Mrs. Fields' mother, and knew that her owner shared the same feeling with her mother. When I told Mrs. Fields that her cat was feeling lonely and ignored, Mrs. Fields began to cry. She felt terrible that her cat was so sad and that she was the reason why. I then told her that the cat told me this was an old issue she shared with her mother. Mrs. Fields was astounded at the cat's insight. Yes, she had felt lonely and abandoned by her mother when she was young. Her mother was a successful lawyer and many times had worked long hours. And why did this problem suddenly emerge with the cat? Mr. and Mrs. Fields were trying to have a baby and were having difficulty. Chula sensed this and knew that Mrs. Fields was not going to get pregnant until she resolved her old hurt and fear of abandoning the baby, the way her mother had abandoned her.

Your desires will also trigger the soul to release buried emotions. Whatever you desire, the soul attracts into your life. If you have a past hurt associated with that desire, the soul will create an incident to show you it. In order to have what you want, you must be prepared to first deal with any old hurts associated with it. See Chapter 15 for more details concerning this.

Unfelt emotions are stored in the chakras in the nadis, the energy arteries within the chakras. Pockets are created to hold the stored emotions. You can picture it like the accumulation of too much cholesterol in your blood arteries. Unfelt emotions create similar blocks in your energy field. And just like a cardiovascular system clogged with too much cholesterol, an energy field clogged with too many unfelt emotions reduces your life force and eventually leads to death. This will appear in your aura like a tear, a gap, or a black area. The longer an unfelt emotion sits in the chakra, the thicker and denser, more physical it becomes. As the emotion gets denser, it begins to leave the chakra and travels into the body's organs then down the meridians to other parts of the body where it begins to manifest itself as a physical ailment, disease or injury.

Some chakras will be blocked more than others. If you look at your body, you can get a good idea which chakras give you more trouble. Look at your torso. The areas where you carry more padding or girth, or where you have a tendency to hold your weight will be the areas where your chakras are blocked. People who are barrel-chested or who have large breasts are people who want to protect their Heart Chakras. People with big stomachs, or people who work out to make their stomachs hard and muscular, are people who feel powerless and want to protect their Solar Plexus Chakras. People who carry their weight in their hips or buttocks have Root Chakra issues.

Also, where do you carry your stress? Chances are, there are old buried hurts that make that part of the body more sensitive. Stress in the lower back means money or career worries. Stress in the stomach means you are feeling powerless to something going on in your life. Stress in the lower intestines, means you are feeling victimized by someone or something. Stress in the back of the neck means you are feeling pressured by too many responsibilities, or by what people are saying. These are just a few generalizations. If you want more information and wish to discover the old hurt causing you to be sensitive in these areas, read the chapters on the chakras regarding this.

There are two ways that the energy of an emotion can be released. The first way is the simplest and that is by feeling the emotion while it is still energy. The second way is after it has become denser, through physical matter such as a malady in the body.

How Your Energy System Creates the Events of Your Future

Your energy system is your future. What lies in your soul and what is buried in your chakras will determine what your future holds. Your energy system will attract to you, people with similar energy to yours. These people will then help you to create the events in your life that will bring you conscious awareness of what lies buried in your chakras and your soul.

Exercise:

I want you to take a moment to think about the energy system of your body.

1. How far do you think your energy system extends beyond your body?
2. When you are standing next to someone, where do you think your energy field ends and the other person's begin?
3. When your energy field comes into contact with someone else's energy field what do you think happens? Do you think the energy fields collide as though they are two walls that slam up against each other? Or do you think the energy fields blend?

I found that when you are standing next to another person, your energy field blends with theirs. When energy fields blend, they speak to each other. They send signals back to the brain. Some times we pick up on these signals and know them as gut feelings or sizing someone up. But most of the time we are oblivious to them. Yet what is said during this exchange many times creates the beginning of a future event.

For example, Mary has an issue with trust. She keeps going out with men who cheat on her. She just met Ron who also has an issue with trust. He knows he can't be trusted. When their energies meet, their souls know it's a perfect match. They are immediately attracted to each other. Mary knows Ron is perfect for her. He won't cheat on her. Ron knows Mary is the right one for him. This time he'll be faithful. But all the time they are together, their souls are speaking to each other through their energy fields. Mary's is saying to Ron, "Cheat on me, cheat on me. It's my learning lesson. It's in my genes. My dad cheated on my mom and you have to do it to me." Ron has the same lesson, and the same genes, his father cheated on his mother. His soul is saying to hers, "Don't trust me. I'm going to cheat on you." Their story goes this way. After being together for a few months, Ron gets antsy and tells Mary he's going out with the guys. In the beginning he does. He and his friends meet once a week and hang out at the local bar. But after a few times, his eyes begin to wander. Ron cheats on Mary. At first he feels guilty, then later resentful, thinking to himself, she deserves it for trusting him and being so gullible thinking he's going out just for drinks. Of course you know how the story ends. Mary finds out Ron has been unfaithful. Ron blames Mary for making him unfaithful. Their souls are crying, "What does it feel like to be cheated on? What does it feel like to be the cheater?"

For Mary this was a painful experience. She finally felt all the emotions of what it feels like to be cheated on. She gave her soul what it wanted. She cried and cried and bemoaned the history of her love life. She stopped dating, knowing she couldn't trust herself with men. Six months later she saw Ron again. Her first reaction was, "What did I ever see in him!" There was no more attraction. It was plain to her now; this man couldn't be trusted. Mary's energy field had changed. She was no longer screaming for someone to cheat on her. Now that she had gained the wisdom, she knew what a cheater felt like and could spot one a mile away.

You don't have to be standing in someone's energy field to start an event. Your soul will do this for you. Your soul knows when a building is going to collapse or a hurricane is going to take place, or a particular stranger is going to run a red light. If your soul feels you need a freak experience to shock you into feeling your emotions, then your soul will make sure you are in the right spot, at the right time to experience it.

Through your seed pattern you will continue to do the same thing over and over. What happened originally in the first eight years will set you up into recreating the event again. This will all be done on a subconscious level, without any conscious awareness. For instance, when Joe was five, he got into a fight with his younger brother, which caused his brother to accidentally bang his head against the coffee table. His brother required stitches. Joe felt guilty about what he did. His father punished him by giving him a severe spanking. Joe's subconscious associated hurting his brother with physically being hurt himself. When Joe became an adult, he continued the subconscious association. Whenever he said or did anything to hurt his brother or someone else, he later created a minor accident to hurt himself. One time it was slamming his finger in a drawer. Another time it was cutting his hand while slicing bread. Joe punished himself because that's what his father taught him: when you hurt others, you hurt yourself. The only way Joe could stop the pattern would be to feel the emotion lying beneath the action.

The Simple 4-Step System

You do not need another physical event to occur to know the lessons buried in your chakras and in your soul. You only need to *remember* your past to know your lessons. The System For Soul Memory will help you to remember. Once you learn more about the chakras and understand their development, you will know where to look for the source of your problems. Once you know the source, The System For Soul Memory will then teach you how to feel them emotionally. Feeling them emotionally will create the shortcut to having a transcendental 'knowing' of them. When you 'know' an emotion while it is still in your subconscious, you will be making your life easier. You will be intervening in the soul's process of having to devise future events to get you to learn your lessons.

The 4 steps in Chapter 4 create this shortcut. It takes your awareness from what is going on outside you to what is going on inside you. It teaches you how to understand your soul and your subconscious. You do this by learning where your emotions reside; then by getting to know what your emotions are and feeling them.

Your emotions reside in all your chakras. As stated previously, each chakra has a theme and a certain grouping of emotions that resonate to that theme. Chapters 5-12 go into depth about each Chakra. These chapters will tell you about the chakras, their themes, and what emotions you will find in them. I am hoping they will trigger a memory of something that may have happened to you.

These chapters will also tell you about some of the physical blocks created from those emotions when they go unfelt. Knowing this should help you figure out your own emotional blocks. Maybe you are suffering from an illness and you are having trouble healing. For example, Bruce has prostate problems. He has no idea what the buried emotion could be that is causing his distress. In reading through the chapters on the various chakras, Bruce discovers that the prostate is associated with the Root Chakra found in Chapter 5. In reading the chapter he discovers that this chakra develops from conception through the age of 1, and that the emotions associated with this chakra deal with security. Bruce can't remember anything about being a baby, but he does remember what his parents told him. He was born at the worst time in their life, when they couldn't afford him, because they were out of work and in debt. Bruce realizes that his own life is reflecting the same issues. He too is struggling to make ends meet. His mortgage is too high, he can't afford his house. He owes the credit card company twenty thousand dollars, and no matter how hard he works, he never has enough. He feels that as a man and husband he is a failure to his wife and family. He can't offer them the security they deserve. These are the emotions Bruce must feel.

Maybe there is a specific aspect in your life you wish to change. For example, Gina sings and is trying to make a career of it. She is having trouble getting jobs. Gina reads the chapters on the chakras and discovers that the Throat Chakra in Chapter 9 is associated with singing. Gina can't remember anything specific that happened to her during the age of five when the Throat Chakra first developed, but she does feel strong emotions every time she thinks about her stalled career. She follows the steps in Chapter 4. Gina discovers she has trouble fully feeling her emotions. Not until she reads Chapter 13 and learns how to feel an emotion fully, is Gina able to finally release them. Once she does this. Gina remembers an incident that occurred when she was five. She wanted to take dance lessons with her friends, but her mother wouldn't let her. Her mother told her that dance lessons were a waste of money and wouldn't do much for her in life. Gina was living her mother's words and proving them true. Subconsciously, she believed that singing, like dancing, was a waste of time and wouldn't do much for her in life.

In each chapter, I ask you questions to make you think about yourself. In thinking about yourself, you may realize the source of your current problems. Hopefully the client stories that follow will help trigger similar blocked emotions in you.

If you have done the four steps and are still stymied about what your blocked emotions are, then Chapter 13 should help. In Chapter 13, I will teach you how to feel your emotions. I will teach you how to think about them in a new way, in terms of energy. It is much easier to feel your emotions when you think about them in this way.

The rest of the chapters will teach you more about energy and the energy system of your body. They will show you some of the subconscious ways energy is used.

I changed the name of the clients in the stories, and in some cases I even changed the stories to make my point as simple and clear as possible. The accuracy of the story is not important. What is important, is that the stories become the vehicle to help trigger and heal the emotional blocks in you. I am hoping that in the stories I tell, you will see a similar pattern happening in you. By the time you are finished reading this book, you should have a much better understanding of yourself.

4

The System for Soul Memory

1. Choose a problem or situation you wish to change. In your mind, recreate the circumstances surrounding it. Visualize it as though you are watching a movie.
2. While you are recreating the situation in your mind, allow all your emotions to surface. Where in your body are you feeling them? Look at Diagram 2 to see which chakra the situation is residing. After identifying which chakra the problem resides, look at Diagram 2 to see at what age the problem first originated. Can you remember a similar incident occurring back then?
3. While thinking about the problem or incident, what is the emotion that surfaces? Name the emotion.
4. Feel the emotion.

These simple four steps comprise the heart of the System For Soul Memory. These simple steps will give the soul what it wants, the transcendental knowing of an event. These steps will enable you to use the past to learn your lessons. You will not need further future events to get you to react, to feel. You will be taking charge of your life by intervening in the soul's process.

In order to do the above exercise properly; you will need time and privacy. I recommend doing the exercise at home in the evenings when you know you will not be disturbed. You cannot allow for any interruptions. No people, no phones, no children, no pets, etc. The purpose of this exercise is to get you to feel your emotions, to make you cry, get angry and upset. In order to fulfill the requirements of transcendence, you must allow yourself to feel intensely. Any interruptions will disturb the flow of energy.

Prepare yourself well for the event. Make this a sacred occasion devoted especially to you. Be consciously aware that you intend to change your life, to heal what is troubling you. Wear comfortable clothing, have a glass of water nearby, and a box of Kleenex. Situate yourself someplace cozy, where you feel safe. If there are people involved in your problem and you have a photograph of them, place it near you. Use whatever props you have that will help you remember the situation clearly. In this exercise, you are going to allow yourself to let go and feel what you normally prevent yourself from feeling.

In this exercise, you will be using the energy system of your body. In other words, you will only be *thinking* and *feeling*. You will not be physical, or acting anything out. You will be internalizing everything. Don't be discouraged if you don't get incredible results the first time you practice this exercise. This just means you are not accustomed to feeling your emotions. I discovered that many people don't know how to feel their emotions. If that is the case, read Chapter 13, and keep practicing. Learning to feel your emotions is like learning to walk, or lift weights. You don't run a marathon or lift a hundred pounds the first time you try.

Step One. Choosing the Problem or Situation You Wish to Change

Choose a situation or a problem you wish to resolve, or change. This can be an event that occurred that is still troubling you, or something in your life that has been a reoccurring problem. This could be anything: a problem at work, at home, in a relationship, how you are treated, etc. The first time you are using the System For Soul Memory, I recommend choosing a problem that brings up strong emotions, a problem that you are still sensitive to. This will help make using the system easier and give you a better understanding of it.

Take a moment to relax. Close your eyes and take three deep breaths. Keep your eyes closed, and recreate the situation in your mind. Picture in your mind a movie screen and watch the events that took place, unfold. See and feel yourself back in the situation.

Step Two. Allowing the Emotions to Surface

Once you are deeply involved in the incident, allow all your emotions to surface. As the emotions begin to surface, be on guard that you don't squelch them or push them away. Allow them the freedom to bloom. Begin to concentrate on them instead of the movie screen. You will notice that these emotions are sitting in a particular spot in your body. Where are they sitting? In your neck, your head, your abdomen, your heart, etc. Look at Diagram 2 to match up that part of the body with the corresponding chakra. The heart belongs to the Heart Chakra; the abdomen to the Solar Plexus Chakra, your belly to the Naval Chakra, etc. Once you have located the chakra, look at Diagram 2 again, and notice at what age that chakra first developed.

Think back to when you were that age. Does one particular incident stand out? Generally the subconscious will bring to mind the correct, corresponding incident. If you can't remember back that far continue to step three. If you can remember the incident, bring it to the movie screen in your mind and play it again as if it were happening now. Allow the emotions to surface. If you followed the steps correctly, you should be feeling the same emotions in the same chakra as you felt for the current situation.

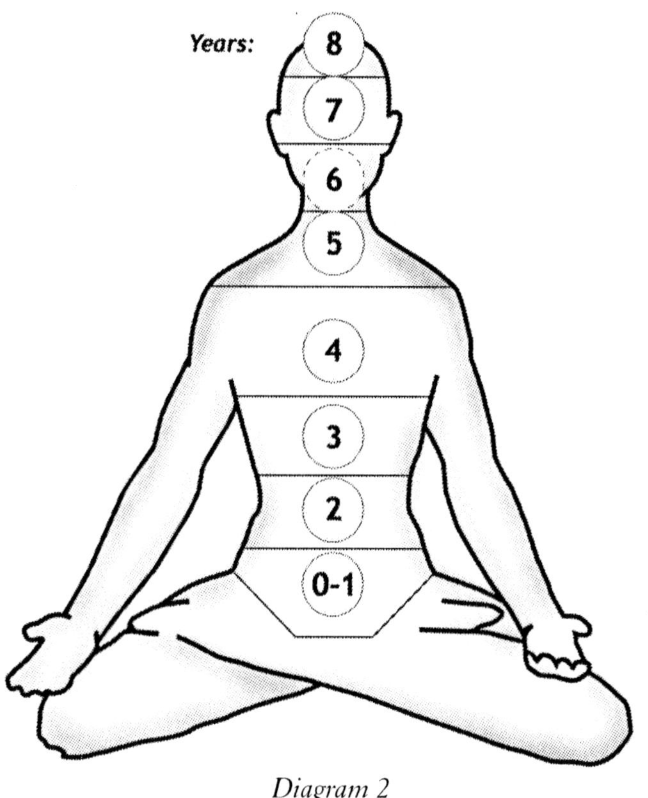

Diagram 2

Once you see and the feel the connection to the past, you should have an instantaneous learning of the emotion. This will feel like a burst of energy, 'a light going off in your head,' like a heavy weight has been lifted from your chest, etc. Transcendence has been reached. When transcendence has been reached and your soul has been given the information it wants, you will know it. Remembering the past, the seed pattern, makes it much easier to learn your lesson. You will not have to go further, and do anymore steps. It is that simple.

If you were not so lucky and made no connection to the past, then you have more work to do. Continue to step three.

Step Three. Naming the Emotion

Bring yourself back to the current situation. Allow your emotions to surface once more. Feel the emotion in the chakra in which it is sitting. What emotion you are feeling? Give it a name. Read Chapter 13 if you are having trouble distinguishing the emotion you are feeling. If you have read the chapter and are still having problems, then continue to focus your attention on whatever you are feeling in the chakra. If you continue to focus your attention on that feeling, even if this takes days or weeks, eventually the emotion will become discernible, and you will know the emotion.

Step Four. Feel the Emotion

Once you know the emotion you are feeling, feel it. Concentrate solely on the emotion. Cry, feel hate, be sad, get angry ... do whatever you must to get yourself deeply involved with the emotion. Feel it intensely. If your concentration slips and you are losing the emotion, replay the movie of the current situation in your mind to once more bring up the emotion. Feel the emotion until there is no more emotion to feel.

Your life will reflect whether or not you have fully felt the emotion. If you have learned the lesson, the situation will no longer bother you or be an issue in your life. The emotional block will be freed from your chakra. Your soul will no longer have to replay similar events in your future.

How the Four Steps Work

Throughout the book I have stated that in order for the soul to gain wisdom, for you to learn your lesson, you must have conscious awareness of your life on a physical, mental, and emotional level. In the first step when you are remembering the situation and creating the movie, you are establishing conscious *physical* awareness of the event.

In the second step, you are asked to remember a similar experience in your childhood by figuring out which chakra the emotion resides and at what age it was first presented. This helps you to remember the seed pattern. It is much easier to feel an emotion when you remember it as a child. This is basically what 'inner child' work is all about. If you can remember the seed pattern, you will learn your lesson much more quickly and easily.

The third step deals with having conscious *mental* awareness of the emotion and the event. In other words, you are concentrating on yourself instead of what is going on outside you. You are realizing that when the event occurred, you acted a particular way, it made you think in a particular way, and in thinking in that particular way, it made you feel a particular emotion. If you think back to when the event first occurred, you were probably so busy reacting to the event, you weren't even aware of you.

The fourth step gives you conscious *emotional* awareness. You do this by feeling the emotion solely, until there is no more emotion to feel. When you complete all four steps, you gain the wisdom the soul seeks. You will have a transcendent knowing of the lesson programmed into your soul.

5

The Root Chakra

Zone 0-1 (Color: Black)

Developmental Age

The Root Chakra develops from the moment of conception through the first year of life. At the moment of conception, the soul takes charge of the body. This is when the soul of the baby overlays with that of the mother's. Not until puberty is this connection severed. Everything that happens in the womb is recorded in the soul, including the thoughts and feelings of the parents.

Developmental Theme

The Root Chakra deals with survival of the self at the expense of everyone else. Think of a baby. In the womb, the baby is a parasite. The baby feeds off the mother's body. After he is born, the baby continues to be self-absorbed and thinks only of having his needs met—how he is sheltered, fed, and cared for. The baby 's concern is one of survival.

About the Chakra

Any kind of trauma or major event that occurred after conception through the first year of life will manifest throughout your life as problems relating to survival. Survival means, the physical aspects of your life: your house, work, food, career, money, prosperity or lack of, and safety. In other words, like a baby, how you are sheltered, fed and cared for. It is hard to remember being one year of age, or even going back further to being in the womb. But the subconscious, the soul, remembers everything. Hypnosis or meditation can help you remember when your seed patterns first occurred. Otherwise, ask parents or family members what they remember.

Also found in the Root Chakra are all issues dealing with male sexuality. In most Chakric literature, you will find both male and female sexuality grouped together in either the Root Chakra or the Naval Chakra. Throughout my ten years of study, of counseling both men and women, I have consistently found male sexuality issues to exist in the Root Chakra, and female sexuality issues to exist in the Naval Chakra. Therefore, that is how you will find it in The System For Soul Memory. As you know men and women are different. Their overall driving force is different. Male energy moves, it is aggressive, action oriented. Female energy receives; it is passive, nurturing and stabilizing. Male is the warrior. Female the negotiator. Look at the body's anatomy to see how this follows. Yet each person regardless of sex, is both male and female. Both energies are found in the body. The male in you keeps you moving, taking action. It wants to be physical, to make things and fix things. It is the part of you that is the aggressor, and that protects you when you are in danger. The female in you wants to nurture and receive, to understand. It is your nesting instinct.

Therefore, for a male, the root chakra is where his sexuality is developed. If you have any problems with impotence, look to the first year of your life for any traumas. Energy blocks in the Root

Chakra can lead to sexual problems such as impotence, or an overactive sex drive. Also if you are male and have issues with your father that are not dealt with, this will show up later as prostate or testicular problems.

Blocked Energy Manifestations

Blocked energy in the Root Chakra manifests through problems in the following areas:

Work
Career
Money Problems
Home
Living situations
Safety
Food Problems – as a physical manifestation where there is starvation or nutritional deficiency
Male sexuality

Emotions

The following emotions are Root Chakra emotions:
Self trust - Feeling safe and secure in your world
Self worth - Feeling worthy enough
Selfishness
Vanity
Lust/sensuality
Passion
Aggression

Possible Health Problems from Energy That Has Been Blocked Too Long

Bladder problems

Male sexuality problems such as impotence or an overactive sex drive
Prostate / testicular problems
Lower back problems
Lower colon and bowel problems
Rectal problems
Some leg, knee, ankle or feet problems[4]

Potential Traumas from the Womb
Questions to Ask Yourself

Were you wanted as a baby? Did your mother ever think of aborting you?

From the moment of conception, the soul begins recording everything. Even how your parents felt. While you are in the womb, your soul feels everything. An unborn baby knows when it is not wanted. If your parents didn't want you, then you will have major problems in life with the emotion of self worth-of having the right to have things. For some people this can also manifest as even having the right to exist.

Example: Sally's mother was upset when she found herself pregnant with Sally. Too much was going on her life at the time and having another child to care for, was the last thing Sally's mother wanted. Sally grew up with this feeling buried deep within her. Most of her life she went out of her way to please her mother, but she found she never could. This blocked emotion manifested as feelings of unworthiness—a low level of "I Deserve." In Sally's life this revealed itself through her career. Sally is an Interior Decorator. Every time her business picks up, it suddenly stops and goes flat. Sally can't seem to do more than break even.

How was the pregnancy? Any health problems? Any birth problems?

Any health problems during pregnancy or with the birth procedure is very traumatic for a baby. This leads to Root Chakra issues later in life.

For example: The umbilical chord choking you, can lead later to a constant feeling of being strangled by life:

Rachel's birth was traumatic. She nearly died when the umbilical chord strangled her during delivery. Her mother had often told her the story. What Rachel didn't realize was its impact on her life. Rachel kept getting jobs that dead-ended, that went nowhere. She couldn't seem to make enough money to move out of her parent's home, to have a home of her own. Whenever she saved enough money to move on, a crisis occurred that consumed the little money she saved. Rachel couldn't seem to get ahead.

Subconsciously, Rachel was still traumatized by her birth. Moving forward through the birth canal, and knowing it as death, left her with the fear of moving forward in life. When I asked Rachel what it would feel like to move out of her parent's house, she panicked and said she was frightened that she would die. To Rachel, those still unresolved but strong emotions are still ruling her life. Not until she goes back and faces those traumatic feelings from birth, will she be free of them.

Potential Problems During the First Year

How was your parent's health? Was there ever a time when your mother was too sick to care for you? Did your parents ever experience an emotional upset?

Having someone else care for you feels like abandonment to the baby. Or if your mother is distracted and not paying close attention to your needs is very upsetting.

Example: John's grandmother died in a freak accident a month after he was born. His mother grieved deeply. She had trouble coming to terms with the sudden loss of her mother. She tried caring for John, but sometimes the grief was too great and she had to farm John out to other family members. John as a baby was too young to understand the abandonment. He was also too young to understand his mother's strong emotions. He took his mother's feelings of loss and made them his own. To this day he still has an irrational fear of losing his mother. John's blocked energy manifested later in his life as sexual impotence.

Where did you sleep? Think of your crib. Was it roomy, safe, cozy? Quiet, or noisy?

Answer these questions and you will have a good idea of what you were taught to expect from your living space. Your immediate physical environment during your first year of life will establish the beliefs and conditions you will seek subconsciously when you get older. For example: If you shared your bed with another sibling, then as you get older, you might feel you don't have the right to have a space of your own.

For example, Frank and Sybil are brother and sister. Because they were born one right after the other, their mother didn't buy another crib. Frank and Sybil shared their bed. This manifested later in life in different ways for each of them. Frank never owned a place of his own. He always rented. And when he did, he sought shelter in areas that were derelict and not safe.

For Sybil, the blocked emotion manifested differently. She was able to have a home of her own, but never her own space in it. There was never a room where she could go to be alone. This also manifested in the office where she worked. She could never understand why she always ended up sharing a desk with someone else.

What happened when you cried for food? Were you picked up and cared for immediately? Or did you have to wait? If you did wait, are you still waiting to have the things you want most in life? And how hard did you have to cry to get your food? Did you have to scream loud or struggle hard to get it?

All these examples condition a baby on how he will act later in life. For example, Anthony was the fourth son, born in a family of six children. Because there was always a lot of excitement going on in his home, he really had to scream to be heard as a baby. Anthony learned early that he would have to struggle hard for the basic necessities in life. Today, Anthony is working two jobs to make ends meet. Until he unblocks those old feelings that come with neglect and struggle, he will continue to believe that nothing comes easy.

Were you bottle-fed or breast-fed?

It is natural for a baby to be breast-fed. Being breast-fed tells the baby that it is okay to be a parasite, to suck off others, to take and receive things for free. Babies that are bottle-fed will struggle with this notion. Later, they may create situations in their lives where they will want to be parasitic, or be taken care of. Maybe it will be a spouse that provides for them, or the government, disability, unemployment, illness, etc.

How were you fed? Were you rushed through your meal because your mother was too busy with other things?

Maybe now you hate to ask people for things because you feel like you are inconveniencing them.

Were you given more food than you wanted, or maybe not enough? Look at what you have materially. Do you have enough to make ends meet? Or, are you always falling short?

Example: Tom always had to finish the food on his plate. Even if he was satiated, he couldn't let anything go to waste. He'd feel too guilty. He learned this early on from his mother. While feeding him, his mother always made sure Tom finished every drop of milk in the bottle. Today, Tom owns very little in life. He only buys the bare necessities, and it is those things he knows he will use. He doesn't know to have the extras.

When you were born, were there other brothers and sisters around? How did they relate to you getting your needs met? Did

they come first? When you cried for food, were they taken care of first?

Example: Jill was the youngest of three children. Because she, her brother and sister were close in age, she learned early that she would have to wait to be cared for until the older siblings were cared for first. Today, Jill is still putting herself at the bottom of her list. She is married and has two children of her own. She has a list of things she wants, but she won't buy herself anything until her children and husband are taken care of first.

What happened to your family during your first year? Did you move? Being uprooted from your home is very traumatic to a baby. Did both your parents work? Did your father or mother have a job that sent them out of town? Not having your parents around feels like abandonment to a baby.

Example: Stan's father was a traveling salesman. When Stan was born, his father wasn't around much. He was always working in distant cities. Today, Stan is married to a woman whose job takes her away from home quite often. Stan hates that she travels so much, but because her salary is vital to the family's welfare, Stan says nothing.

During the year when you were one, were there any violent weather conditions or natural disasters?

Example: George was visiting California when he was one. Unfortunately, during his stay, he experienced a major earthquake. When George finished graduate school, he moved to California to set up a private practice as a family counselor and therapist. In George's deep subconscious, California represented a place of feeling powerless. Because the earthquake occurred when George was one, George's sense of powerlessness showed itself in his career. Today, George has a hard time making enough money in his practice to support himself and his family.

6

Navel Chakra
Zone 2 (Color: Red)

Developmental Age

The Navel Chakra develops through the second year of life.

Developmental Theme

Just as the Root Chakra deals with survival, so too does the Navel Chakra. Only the Naval Chakra deals with everyone else's survival at your expense. At two years of age a baby becomes aware that other people exist. During this time, the baby learns that others have needs too. How far a baby will go to fulfill the needs of others depends on the circumstances in the baby's life and on the baby's genetic background. This is the time when the baby learns what he must do to satisfy others in order for his own needs to be met. In doing so, the baby learns how to make decisions and how to cooperate with his environment.

About the Chakra

The Root Chakra deals with survival issues that manifest through physical circumstances; in other words, how you will be sheltered, fed, clothed and provided for. The Navel Chakra also deals with survival issues, but on a more emotional and psychological level; in other words, how you *feel and think* about the way you are sheltered, fed, clothed and provided for. Some books written about the chakras call the Navel Chakra the emotional center. As you have read so far, the System For Soul Memory presents *every* chakra as an emotional center. The Navel Chakra is only an emotional center in how it relates to the emotional and psychological issues dealing with *survival*. This is the chakra where you will harbor feelings of being victimized; where you will blame and resent others for hurting you or for not taking good enough care of you, or for not loving you.

Both the Root Chakra and Navel Chakra are the only two chakras dealing mainly with how you exist. They work closely together in how you approach your environment and life. The energy of the Root Chakra is aggressive, warrior-like and allows you take care of yourself. The energy of the Navel Chakra is passive and wants others to care of you.

The Adrenal Gland is associated with this chakra. This gland releases the hormone Epinephrine (adrenaline), which is released when the brain warns us of danger. When we are warned of danger, we have a choice, either to stand and fight, or to flee. The Navel Chakra works closely with the Root Chakra in determining which action you take. The Root Chakra is your male side where you stand and fight. The Navel Chakra, because it is concerned with everyone else's survival at your expense, wants you to flee.

For a female, the Navel Chakra is where her sexuality is developed. If you have any female problems—problems with menstruation, the ovaries, cervix, breasts, getting pregnant, etc—look back to the age of two to see if there were any traumas. Also, if you are a woman and have any resentment or hate for your mother, it will show up as an energy block in this chakra.

Blocked Energy Manifestations

Any kind of trauma or major event that occurred in your life during the age of two will manifest as problems in the following areas:

Codependency issues
Laying blame
Making decisions
Isolation – Feeling lonely, not having enough attention
Emotional and Psychological Food Problems
Female Problems

Emotions Found in This Chakra

Loneliness
Feeling isolated
Craving seclusion
Feeling unsupported
Feeling violated
Feeling attacked
Feeling victimized
Feeling like you are not getting enough attention
Feeling smothered from too much attention
Feeling nurtured/ lack of nurturing
Empathy
Feeling the urge to help others
Feeling like a martyr
Feeling like you are making a sacrifice
Bitterness
Feeling insecure
Feeling unsatisfied, like you will never have enough

Possible Health Problems from Energy That Has Been Blocked Too Long

- Kidney problems
- Adrenal gland problems
- Female problems:
  - Amenorrhea
  - Fibroids
  - Menstrual Problems
  - Vaginitis
  - Cysts, tumors
  - Breast cysts, tumors
  - Problems conceiving
  - Problems with pregnancy
  - Ovaries
- Intestinal problems
- Weight problems, being too fat or too thin
- Eating disorders
- Lower back problems
- Some leg, feet or ankle problems[5]

Questions to Ask Yourself

Did any traumas happen to you during the age of two?

Were you or anyone in your family sick, or in any accidents? Did anyone die? Did you experience any unusual weather conditions or earth changes? Did you move? Did you take a trip? Did your parents experience any unusual stresses? Was a sibling born? If any trauma happened to you during the age of two, it would affect you later in life in the above areas.

How did your mother love you? Were you born to fill a void in her life? Was she feeling unloved?

This is where codependency first originates, where the role of caretaker first begins. If there is any history of addiction in your family, this is when you first sense it as a baby. A baby senses all the mother's feelings. If the mother is feeling unloved in her life, a baby will know this and try to make up for it. The mother's feeling of neediness will have a compulsive attitude. A baby learns to connect this feeling of neediness with its own survival. That's why later, when the baby grows up and gets into a destructive, codependent relationship, he or she might feel their basic survival is at stake if they or the other person walk away.

When you were two, how much attention did you receive?

At two, a baby begins to socialize, to know there are others who exist in the world. How much time were you given for this? Think back to what it was like in your family. Did you come from a big family where there were older siblings who played with you and took care of you? Or were you frequently left alone? If you were frequently left alone, do you often find yourself alone today yet crave to be more social but have trouble accomplishing this.

How about the opposite? Do you crave seclusion but find you are never left alone?

Also, how much attention you received will determine your weight. I have found that people who receive too much attention will be on the thin side. People, who get too little attention, will be on the heavy side. This attention will filter down to how people eat. People who pay too much attention to what they eat and how they eat it will be thin. They generally eat slowly; aware of their bodies, their stomach, and every mouthful they swallow.

People who pay little attention to what they eat and how they eat it, will be heavy. These people like to talk, read or watch TV while they eat. They will look for some kind of outside distraction to take their attention away from their stomachs and their bodies.

The extreme in both these cases will cause eating disorders. This is the chakra where weight problems first develop.

At what age were you taken off the bottle or breast, and given milk to drink from a cup?

When a baby is being fed from the breast or the bottle, the baby is being held. The baby can feel the mother's body, her love and support. When the bottle is taken away and the baby must drink from a cup, the baby will feel a tremendous loss of love. To the subconscious, this transition feels like a trauma. Depending at which age this happens will depend on how it plays out in the baby's life. At one, this trauma will affect the Root Chakra. At two, this trauma will affect the Navel Chakra. To see how it may later affect the baby, read the 'Blocked energy manifestation' concerning each chakra.

At what age were you potty-trained?

Potty training can be traumatic. If you are constipated today, or have stomach problems, or have trouble going to the bathroom, try and remember what happened when you were potty-trained. A traumatic occurrence could cause you to have these problems today.

Knowing your parents today, what do you think you had to do to get attention as a baby? Did you have to be bad, be good, be noisy, and follow the rules?

Example: Elizabeth's mother worked. Elizabeth spent most of her days in a Day Care facility with different babysitters caring for her. The babysitters came and went and gave her little emotional support. Elizabeth learned early that if she was a good, well-behaved baby—in other words, if she didn't cry and complain, but waited patiently— the babysitters did a better job of taking care of her and fulfilling her physical needs. The same followed at home with her busy Mom. Today, Elizabeth is a great mother and wife. She makes sure her kids get more attention and emotional support than she got when she was a child. Even with a full time job, she manages to do everything for her husband and two kids. She is what you would call a Super Mom, and proud of it. Elizabeth's problem today is that she is fighting breast cancer. But that hasn't slowed her down much. Even with the chemotherapy and feeling sick, Elizabeth is still trying to be good and do everything herself. Only that's what's killing her. Elizabeth doesn't know how to ask for help and emotional support. She learned at a very early age that asking for help was a useless endeavor. Until she heals the buried hate she carries from feeling lonely and unsupported, she won't heal. Elizabeth didn't receive the proper nurturing when she was a baby. What Elizabeth must learn now is how to nurture herself. She must learn to pay more attention to herself, and make herself top priority in her life.

Was all of your parent's attention focused on you?

When you received attention from your parents, was there someone else around that interfered? Were you taught to share attention? In other words, when your parent was holding you or playing with you, did you have another brother or sister around, or even another relative, getting in the way, detracting your parent's attention away from you? Look at your life today. Is there a third party interfering with your relationships? Does your spouse spend more time with his/her friends than you? Do parents or in-laws get in the way of your relationship? How much attention are you willing to receive? If you find yourself receiving too much attention, do you subconsciously bring in someone else to take "all that" attention away from you?

Was the attention you received, positive or negative? When you cried or complained too much how did your parents respond? Were they allowing or did they punish you?

Look at how you receive attention today and that will tell you how you were treated as a baby. When you receive attention today, what happens? If you received emotional abuse or criticism as a child are you still getting that kind of attention today? Or how about physical punishment? If you were spanked or hit a lot as a child, are you subconsciously still doing that to yourself today? The self-abuse might show up as being too prone to accidents.

Did you receive more attention in a social setting than at home?

If you did, you'll love being social. Your subconscious comfort level of being with people will have first started at this time. How are you with groups? Would you rather be out than being at home? Look back and see where that belief first started. If you are a loner now, were you frequently left alone? If so, you will be more comfortable today being alone.

When you were two and crying because you were feeling lonely, how did your mother or the person caring for you respond?

Picture yourself being two again. You are lying in the crib. You are feeling lonely. You cry. How does your mother respond?

Example: Stan has a weight problem. Stan's mother has a weight problem too. When Stan was a baby, every time he cried from the crib, his mother automatically assumed it was because he was hungry. Being a food lover, she never imagined that he just wanted to be held. She would play out her genetic disposition to being fat. She would give Stan food and if he refused, she would put him back in the crib or the playpen, not even suspecting that Stan was lonely and wanted company. Stan wasn't receiving enough attention. He learned quickly that the only way he would receive companionship was to eat. He began to associate food with comfort and love. Today, when Stan feels lonely, he goes to the refrigerator to eat. If he felt the emotion instead of acting it out, Stan would no longer have a weight problem.

Was there a time when you were sick or had an accident where you, as a helpless baby, thought you might die?

Amazingly, every person I have counseled who is obese today has had an incident at the age of two when they thought they might die. People who carry a lot of weight on a subconscious level want to be noticed; they need the attention, even if it is negative. This is done for survival reasons. If they are big enough, people will pay attention to them. If people are watching them, and something happens, then they have a better chance of surviving.

Example: Sherry was two when she developed a bad cold. Her parents didn't pay enough attention to her to realize that the cold had gotten worse. It wasn't until Sherry's aunt came to visit that she noticed Sherry was burning with fever. She was the one who suggested that Sherry be rushed to the hospital. That act saved Sherry's life. Sherry had developed pneumonia.

This trauma and the unfelt feelings of helplessness and loneliness didn't show up again in Sherry's life until she became a mother herself. When her child turned two, Sherry suddenly came down with a case of bronchitis that wouldn't heal. She became very depressed and couldn't understand why she felt so lonely and sad. She put on a tremendous amount of weight. When her two-year-old child developed a cold, she became irrationally concerned, checking his crib every few minutes to make sure he was still alive. It wasn't until Sherry remembered her own incident, that she was able to understand her actions and emotions.

7

Solar Plexus Chakra Zone 3 (Color: Orange Red)

Developmental Age

The Solar Plexus Chakra develops during the age of three.

Developmental Theme

The Solar Plexus Chakra deals with power issues. This is a time when a child becomes interested in exploring more of his world. What happens during this year of life will determine how powerful he will feel later in life.

About the Chakra

In Eastern traditions, the Solar Plexus is the seat of Chi. Through meditation, I learned that chi is spiritual energy. It is the energy we receive from God through our souls. When energy is taken into the body it is stored in the Solar Plexus Chakra where it is then directed to other parts of the body.

Energy is taken into the body in different ways. One way the body receives energy is from the soul. The soul sends us energy in the form of our emotions. The next time you feel a rush of emotion, pay attention to how it feels. You will notice how powerfully it exerts itself. If you allow yourself to feel the emotion, you will increase the level of energy in your body. I witnessed this many times in the auras of people who were crying or feeling strong emotion. Their aura's doubled to twice their normal size and glowed with bright color and light.

Eastern religions believe energy is also received from the air we breathe in the form of prana. Prana is to chi what oxygen is to blood. According to Swami Muktananda, prana is "life-breath, the vital force which sustains life and is the power of animation."[6] That is why many Yogis practice deep breathing exercises. They consider prana to be a very powerful healing tool and meditation tool, creating good health and spiritual insight. In terms of energy, think of it as subatomic energy, the 'consciousness of God' found in the air we breathe.

There are also other ways in which we receive energy. One way is from the people around us. In Eastern tradition, devout followers will sit at the feet of their Gurus to receive spiritual energy called *Shaktipat.* Once again, according to Swami Muktananda, "There are four different ways in which *Shaktipat* can be received: *Sparsha diksha*, through the Guru's physical touch; *mantra diksha*, through his words; *drik diksha*, through his look; *manasa diksha*, through his thought."[7] I found that you don't need a guru to transmit energy to you. We are doing it to each other all the time. If you pay attention to the people around you, observe who makes you feel good and who drains you. Those people that make you feel good are people who are sending you energy. Those people who drain you are stealing energy from you. I call these people energy vampires. Energy vampires are people who won't feel their emotions. In not allowing themselves to feel their emotions, they restrict the flow of energy from the soul causing their life force to be weak. Because their life force is weak, they are desperate for energy and will steal it from wherever they can. Any time you feel tired after being around someone, you know you have been in the presence of an energy vampire.

A fourth way of receiving energy is from our environment, from nature. Put your arms around a tree if you need some extra energy or healing. Sit before the ocean, or on a mountain, or in the snow. Anytime you sit in nature, you are being fed energy. Many indigenous civilizations have known this for centuries. Look at their sacred sites and you will find areas of great power.

Animals are also sources of energy. I found them to be great healers. Especially pets. I have encountered this repeatedly in my counseling sessions as a pet psychic. Pets know how to adjust themselves to your energy. They know when you are stressed or feeling sad, and will act like sponges to take the stress or sadness away from you. Take for example the case of Peter the Parrot. Georgia came to me one day complaining that Peter wouldn't stop biting her. She noticed it happened when her boyfriend was around. Once I communicated with the parrot I heard a different story. The parrot told me that Georgia became stressed and unhappy whenever she was around her boyfriend. So Peter did what parrots do when they fear danger, they bite their loved one to warn them and protect them. When I told Georgia this, she was shocked. She didn't want to believe it. But in talking to her further, she saw how she was unhappy in her relationship. She later realized why she was in a state of denial. She was afraid of failing in another relationship. Three weeks later Georgia and Peter came for a visit. Georgia told me Peter was much happier and so was she. She threw out her boyfriend and life was better.

The Solar Plexus Chakra is where energy is stored and directed to other parts of the body. The glands and organs found in Solar Plexus chakra are the stomach, the liver, the spleen, and the pancreas. These glands and organs also send nourishment to the rest of the body.

Blocked Energy Manifestations

Any kind of trauma or major event that occurred in your life during this year will manifest later as feeling powerless, generally in that particular area where the trauma occurred. For example, if at the age of three you experienced an earthquake, then throughout your life you will feel powerless to the earth or to the location where the earthquake occurred. If at the age of three your parents got a divorce, then later in life you will feel powerless to love. If at the age of three your parents moved, then you will feel powerless to new living conditions or situations, etc. etc.

Also, if you suffer from allergies, look back to a situation that made you feel powerless and notice the environment or the foods that were present when the situation occurred. For instance, Tom was driving on a slick, rain swept road when his car veered out of control and crashed into a tree. After the incident, Tom developed an allergy to tree pollen. Terri was eating popcorn at the movies when a man sitting behind her, tried to grope her. Terri later developed an allergy to corn. Or take the case of Phil. He was eating lobster with his girlfriend in a restaurant when she told him their relationship was over. Phil later developed an allergy to fish.

When you discover the incident where your allergy first began, you will be able to heal the allergy by re-experiencing the incident and feeling all the emotions that arose.

Emotions

Anger
Hopelessness
Despair
Feeling powerless
Feeling like a failure
Depression
Feeling pessimistic
Discouraged
Disheartened
Apathy
Feeling stymied, stonewalled

Feeling defeated
Feeling frustrated

Possible Health Problems from Energy That Has Been Blocked Too Long

Liver problems
Stomach problems
Pancreas problems
Gallbladder problems
Spleen problems
Ulcers
Diabetes
Hypoglycemia
Allergies
Middle back problems
Some knee, leg, feet or ankle problems[8]

Questions to Ask Yourself

At the age of three, were there any traumas in your life?

Did you move? Anyone die? Were any of your sisters or brothers born at this time? Any major earth changes or weather storms? Were you in any car accidents? Did your parents leave home for any reason even for a vacation? What was your parent's work situation? Were you sick? Did you go to the hospital? Did you take any trips? If there was any kind of trauma at this age it would show up in your life as feeling powerless to the cause of that particular trauma.

Example: Gail was the oldest of an old fashioned family where the father ruled. Her father's greatest joy and desire was to have many sons. When Gail was born, her father was disappointed. When Gail was three, her father's wish finally came true and her brother was born. Gail immediately sensed the change in the way her father treated her. Gail always felt her father liked her brother better. When Gail was twelve, her mother died. It wasn't until Gail was married and had a son of her own, that problems began to emerge. She was working for a male-dominated chemical firm when suddenly she found she couldn't please her boss. She was fearful she would lose her job to a younger man who started working there six months before. It wasn't until we spoke, and Gail remembered her past, that she was able to make the connection. The emotions were the same. When her brother was born, she was valued less because she was a girl. She could never gain her father's approval the way her brother could. In a similar manner, her boss reminded her of her father. Because work was so male dominated, she felt powerless and left out. In looking back on her life, Gail realized how often she had repressed her feminine side to be more like a man, thinking this would help her gain her father's approval. Once Gail realized this, she quit her job. She no longer desired to repress her feminine side; nor did she need to prove she was just as good as a man by working in such a male dominated field.

Look at your life today. Are there any areas where you feel powerless? Notice those actions you take to feel more powerful.

Examples: These examples are only generalizations and are meant to get you thinking about your own life and what you do to avoid the feelings of powerlessness.

If you are compulsive in lifting weights, taking karate or do anything in relation to self-defense, you are feeling powerless physically, or feeling powerless to your environment. Look back to your childhood. Did someone beat you, or threatened you? Did someone make you feel insecure? Did you live in a bad neighborhood where you felt threatened?

If you spend too much time on your looks, how you dress, your hair, etc., then you are feeling powerless to your body and how you appear to others. This is especially true if you can't be seen in public without being dressed to the max. Also, sometimes, I find people, especially teenagers, who dress like tough guys, wear long hair, outlandish hairstyles, or dress to the extreme with studs, ear piercing, tattooing, or wild makeup, are people who are trying to look tough to hide their extreme sensitivity.

If you spend too much time studying, or reading books, trying to always learn something new, or trying to better yourself, you are feeling powerless to your intelligence. Look around at the people in your life and see who made you feel mentally inferior. For example, by the time Ellen was forty, she had three masters from three different colleges. She always laughed that she was a lifetime student. One of her masters was in social work, so Ellen knew why she was compulsive about school. To the day he died, her father was quick to tell her that because she was a woman, she was mentally inferior. He claimed that the true geniuses in history were always men, like Aristotle, Plato, Newton, and Einstein. Ellen never had her father's approval. Instead of feeling powerless to her father's prejudice, Ellen continued to act out the emotion by going to school and learning more.

Have you ever had any problems with the law, the government or any large institution?

Generally, the law, government or any large institution will represent a strong, powerful, sometimes overbearing figure from your childhood. I found this to generally be the father, or a father-type figure. Many times I counseled people with strong father issues, who, because they loved their parent too much, would instead attract an incident with the law, the government or large institution to work their issue through. It was easier feeling powerless to the law than realizing they felt powerless to their father.

Also, notice the times you get stopped for a traffic violation. Try to remember what you were thinking about, or what event happened just before you were stopped. Chances are you were feeling powerless. Your soul gave you the traffic ticket to make you stop and notice.

For example: Jeffrey was stopped by a policeman and given a traffic ticket for speeding. Jeffrey was very angry and felt he didn't deserve the ticket since he was travelling the same speed as the other cars next to him. Everyone was speeding, yet they didn't get stopped. In talking to Jeffrey, once he was able to pinpoint and feel the emotion, he realized it was the same emotion he was experiencing at work with his boss. He called me later to let me know what happened. After feeling all of his emotions, Jeffrey went back to work. Immediately, his boss's attitude changed. He starting treating Jeffrey better, without Jeffrey saying anything. Just by feeling his emotions, Jeffrey changed the situation at work. He was amazed. Weeks later, Jeffrey had proof again how he had changed his life by feeling his emotions. When he appeared in traffic court to fight the traffic ticket, the judge dismissed it.

Do you suffer from depression?

If you do, then you are not feeling your emotions. They are being repressed to the point where they are affecting the quality of your life. Begin to think about your emotions. Learn why you are not feeling them. Are you feeling powerless to them? I found that feeling powerless to your emotions is a genetic trait that gets reinforced by one of your parents as you grow up. One of your parents made you afraid to feel your emotions. Look back to your childhood to see how this belief was reinforced. How did your parent make you afraid to feel? What did they say or do that gave you this fear? Was someone in your family too emotional or unstable?

How do you handle your anger?

When you get angry what do you do? What did your parents do? Do you react the same way they did, or do you do the opposite because of the hurt their anger caused?

Example: Ira's parents yelled when they got angry. Ira hated it, because it seemed his parents were always yelling. Ira was very intelligent and grew up to be a doctor. He never yelled. In fact he spoke very softly. He spoke so softly, many times people had to lean in closer to hear him. Or they asked him to repeat what he said. Subconsciously, in manipulating people in this manner, Ira felt more powerful.

Ira also learned how to funnel his anger through reasoning and rationalization. In other words, Ira didn't feel his anger, he *buried* it. When he was 65, Ira developed liver cancer and died.

For more information on how to feel anger, look to Chapter 13.

Do you often feel frustrated?

If something frustrates you, then you are feeling powerless to it. Look at your life and see what frustrates you.

Example: Jodi always ran late. It wasn't until her boss mentioned that she wanted to see her at work on time that Jodi made a concerted effort to be early. Her efforts failed. No matter how much time she gave herself, something would happen to make her late. Jodi became frustrated that she couldn't change her habit. In talking with Jodi, she was able to realize the source of her habit. It all began with her mother. When Jodi was younger she fought with her mother when she had to get up and go to school. In looking back, Jodi saw how it was all a power play. Jodi felt powerless to her mother and being late was her way of gaining power over her mother. Jodi then realized that her boss reminded her of her mother. She was just as hardheaded and wouldn't listen to her suggestions, making Jodi feel powerless. Being late was her subconscious means of gaining power over her boss, just as it had been for gaining power over her mother.

8

The Heart Chakra Zone 4 (Color: Blue)

Developmental Age

The Heart Chakra develops during the age of four.

Developmental Theme

The Heart Chakra deals with all issues relating to love.

About the Chakra

At four years old, a child learns what love is. He learns from watching the love in his immediate environment, in his home. He learns about love from his parents, how they interact and love each other, and how they love him.

Think back to the first eight years of your life and remember the way your parents loved each other, and how they loved you. This will tell you what you learned about love. If you liked the example your parents set, then you will follow in their footsteps. If you thought their love was faulty, then you will try to love in a different way.

In spiritual terms, the soul knows that love sustains life. Therefore, the soul wants to know what feels like love and what doesn't. The soul knows that the more we love, the better we live. It is not surprising then, that found in the Heart Chakra, are the heart and the lungs, our main sustainers of life.

Besides the heart and the lungs, the thymus gland is also associated with this chakra. This gland deals with the immune system. It is interesting to note that when the body is being invaded by an organism, the immune system kicks in. Your energy system is the first to feel this invasion on an emotional level. If you suddenly come down with a virus or infection or a disease that affects your immune system, look at your life and see if there was someone or something that you feel invaded your space. This could be a stranger who was too antagonistic, a lover who was too smothering or controlling, a boss who was 'on your case,' a situation that required too much attention, or too many things coming at you once, pulling you in too many directions.

Blocked Energy Manifestations

Any kind of trauma or event occurring during this age will manifest in problems relating to love and relationships.

Emotions

Self Love
Compassion, the love you have for others
Feeling grateful
Abandonment
Betrayal
Rejection
Joy
Sadness
Desire

Mistrust
Yearning/ longing
The feeling of unrequited love
The emotional pain of hurting the ones you love

Possible Health Problems from Energy That Has Been Blocked Too Long

Lung problems
Heart problems
Blood or blood vessel problems
Upper back problems
Immune System problems

Questions to Ask Yourself

At the age of four, were there any traumas in your life?

Did you move? Anyone die? Were any of your sister or brothers born? Any major earth changes or weather conditions? Were you in any car accidents? Did your parents leave home for any reason even for a vacation? Did your parents fight or get divorced? Was your parent's work situation stable? Were you or anyone else sick? Did you take any trips, have any accidents, witness anything traumatic? If anything traumatic happened to you during this age it would affect you later in your relationships, how you love others and how they love you.

How did your parents love each other?

How your parents treated each other will teach you how to love someone else. Did they treat each other with respect? Were they abusive? Did they communicate well? Were they affectionate? Were they generous, self-serving, sacrificing, committed, or responsible? Were they happy, depressed, bitter, or always laying blame? Did they spend a lot of time together, seek each other's company, or were they always out with others?

When you were a child, how did your parents love you?

How your parents loved you, trained you in what to expect in the way others love you. Did your parents treat you with respect? Did they abuse you? Did they treat you as an equal? Did they listen to you? Were they affectionate? Were they generous, selfish, sacrificing? Were they responsible and caring? Did they make you feel special? Did they spend enough time with you? Were they happy to be with you?

Did your parents divorce?

If your parents were divorced then chances are you will be confused as to what love is. Divorce means that the way your parents loved each other didn't work. Therefore, what they showed you and taught you by example is a love that hurts and leads to failure. Since their example of love failed you, you won't know what kind of love works.

I also found in working with people, that if your parents never dealt with the emotions that caused their divorce, then chances are you didn't either. When your parents were divorced, they divorced you too. Divorce is painful for the entire family and feels like a death to the soul: the death of the family, the death of the love you knew growing up. The soul requires a mourning period. All the emotions involved must be felt, whether they are rejection, abandonment, failure or betrayal.

Did your parents have a strong marriage, but you are now having trouble with relationships?

If your parents truly had a strong marriage then you will have no problem having a good marriage too. But don't get confused by what *looks* good. Being married for many years, never fighting, being responsible, being considerate, and committed, does not make the marriage a happy and strong one. Many times a marriage looks right, but doesn't feel right. If you shun love, intimacy, have no desire for a relationship, or are having trouble being in a relationship today, then something was wrong with your parent's relationship. Generally, there was hidden pain. Your subconscious will know and remember this pain, and prevent you from having a satisfactory relationship. If your parents buried their emotions, then you have a good chance of having learned how to bury yours too.

Example: Bill and Alice Leonard were married for 42 years and had three children. Everyone said they had a good marriage up until the day he died of a heart attack. Their children's love life manifested this way: Angela, the oldest, is working on her third marriage. Doug, the middle child, is working on his second; while, Jonathan, the youngest, never married. This is a good example of a dysfunctional marriage that affected the children.

Did one of your parents cheat?

If one of your parents was unfaithful and did not deal with the emotions involved, then you will be unfaithful or be in a relationship where cheating occurs. To the soul, cheating is very painful. Even if you are in an open relationship and give each other permission to fool around, the soul still feels the pain. Not until you feel the pain of hurting the one you love, will you stop the desire to be unfaithful.

Do you now get into relationships where there's a third party?

Do you find yourself in a relationship where you feel your lover spends more time or cares more for someone else rather than you? The third party can be another lover, an ex, even a dead lover, a parent, another family member, a child, or friend. If you feel this way in your relationship, then look back to the first eight years of your life and see how your parents loved you. You learned back then how to be in a triangle relationship. Did one of your parents play favorites with another sibling? Did one of your parents spend more time with their family or friends rather than with you, making you feel like you came second?

For example, Jim complained that his wife was too close to her family. He resented that she spent too much time with them. He felt left out, especially when something happened and she ran to them for help instead of to him. In talking to Jim, he realized he learned this type of love from his mother. His father was a hard, strict man. Whenever there was a problem, his mother ran to her family for love and comfort. She found little love from his father. In talking to Jim further, he realized that on a deep subconscious level he was asking his wife to run to her family for support. Jim didn't know how to give her the support himself. He was never taught. Once Jim realized this, he began to cry. He saw how he was never supported as a child, and could feel the old buried pain. Afterwards, Jim's relationship changed. He and his wife became closer.

Does your lover keep a part of his/her heart from you?

Look back and remember the way your mother and father loved each other. Was their love so strong you felt excluded?

Did one of your parents lose a lover before they married that they never finished mourning? Or a child? If your parents closed their hearts because they didn't want to feel their pain, then this would feel like a loss of love for you. Later in life you would be attracted to this kind of love, someone who keeps a part of his or her heart closed off. Again, this is the kind of love you knew growing up; therefore, you will feel the most comfortable with it.

Take the case of Lila. She married Gil, a widower whose wife died young of breast cancer. When Lila married Gil, she knew he still carried a torch for his dead wife. Gil kept pictures of her everywhere. In the beginning of their marriage, Lila thought Gil would eventually change. She thought that being married to her would be enough to make him happy, so that he would forget his dead wife. After three years nothing changed. Lila felt like there was a ghost getting in the way of her marriage. This was the situation when Lila came to see me. I asked Lila if she remembered anything similar happening to her parents; did either one lose a lover before they married. She related how her father had been married before he met her mother, but the wife was still living. She knew this because her father was always calling the ex-wife, and her mother was always complaining about it. As soon as Lila said this she saw the connection to her own life. She saw how she felt rejected by her father because she sensed that he loved his ex-wife more than he loved her or her mother. This was the same with Gil. She felt that Gil loved his dead wife more than he loved her. As soon as Lila realized this, she began to cry and heal the old buried pain. Lila called me the following week to let me know what happened. Lila never mentioned our conversation to Gil. Yet three days later, she saw Gil take the pictures he kept around the house of his dead wife and store them in a box in the closet. When she asked Gil why he was doing that, he told her that it was time to bury the past and move on.

Do you feel your lover doesn't support you?

When you were a child and complained to your parents about something someone else did to you, how did they respond? Did they listen to you, believe you, commiserate with you, be on your side, and try to help you? Or did they take a contrary position, explain logically why the other person did what they did, or tell you that you deserved what you got? Does your lover react the same way now, making you feel unsupported?

When you were a child, was one of your parents or a sibling, ill or physically disabled?

If this is the case, examine your role in your relationship with your lover now. How did growing up with someone who was sick or disabled affect the way you love or are being loved today?

If you grew up with someone who was disabled, how much of a caretaker did it make you? Are you that way today? Did you receive less attention growing up because of it? Are you still jealous or resentful because you felt like you were loved less? Or did it make you feel more compassionate?

As a child, because someone at home was sick or disabled, was more responsibility forced on you? Look at your relationship today. Do you feel you are the one forced to carry more of the burdens and responsibilities?

Are you in love with someone today who is always getting sick? Look back to your childhood and see who was always getting sick while you were growing up? If you grew up with a sick person, then subconsciously you will attract this type of person to love. Your soul will attract someone with this type of energy, even though it may not be apparent when you first fall in love. For example, Joanna had a father who suffered with a heart condition. Growing up, she always remembers emergencies where he would be rushed to the hospital. He died when she was twenty. It wasn't until after she married that Joanna learned that her husband suffered from juvenile diabetes. He didn't tell her beforehand, because he claimed he didn't know how. Yet loving a sick man felt normal to Joanna. She never regretted her marriage, even when he died young at the age of forty.

Was one of your parents abusive, whether it was emotional, physical, sexual or from substance abuse?

If you learned this type of love in your childhood, then you will have a difficult journey. When you become an adult, you will want to repeat the abuse you learned as a child. Changing this pattern will be very difficult since it is not only genetic, but also found deep in the soul. Generally, I find people who carry this type of learning lesson want to punish themselves on a deep soul level. Yet those who manage to overcome the difficulties and feel the emotional pain, turn out to be the most compassionate and spiritual people I meet.

There are so many emotions involved in healing abuse, that I always recommend getting help from a qualified agency or counselor. Learning to feel your emotions will have many painful and fearful attachments and will not be easy. Also, training yourself not to act out feelings or be dependent on something physical will take strong determination and patience. Having a professional to support you through the process will be important.

Did the love you receive in your childhood feel stable, or was there constant chaos?

Look at the type of love you receive now. Is it calm, reliable and stable? Or are you, or your mate, constantly creating situations that put you in chaos? Is there much yelling, arguing? Do you find you or your mate being self-destructive and putting yourselves in jeopardy? This could be through money, illness, abuse, etc. Observe yourself. If things get too calm in your love life, do you look for ways to create excitement? If as a child, you were loved in a chaotic environment, then you will look for the same type of relationship when you get older.

Did one of your parents travel away from home a lot? Or did one of your parents live somewhere else?

If this is the case, look at your life now and see if you have learned to love from a distance. Some people feel comfortable having their mate away for long periods of time.

Or are you experiencing the opposite, hating the fact that your mate is away so much? Look to your childhood and see where you learned to love this way. Maybe one of your parents left and there was negativity surrounding his or her departure. Or maybe you were forced to live away from home.

Another case I've seen deals with a mate who travels and invariably, after they go something traumatic happens. This could leave you feeling abandoned and unsupported.

Example: When Esther was four years old, her parents took a trip to Europe, leaving her at home with her grandparents to baby sit. While her parents were away, Esther was bitten by a bee and had a terrible allergic reaction. Later in life, whenever she felt abandoned, she immediately had an allergic reaction to something in her environment. Esther thought she was just sensitive and highly allergic, until she realized the connection between her seed pattern and the emotion of abandonment. Once she realized this and felt the abandonment, her allergic reactions ceased.

How much did your parents hug you? Were they cuddly and touched you frequently? Or were they distant and reserved?

How much physical nurturing do you receive today? Are you satisfied? If not, look back to the past. Again, how your parents loved you whether it was physical or emotional, will be the way you receive love today. If you look back and remember your parents being more physically nurturing than your mate is today, then think back and see if there was one particular incident that was negative that makes you not want to be nurtured today. Remember, your subconscious is telling your mate not to be physical with you. If there is buried emotional pain surrounding the act of being physical, you will not want yourself to be nurtured.

9

The Throat Chakra Zone 5 (Color: Green)

Developmental Age

The Throat Chakra develops during the age of five.

Developmental Theme

The Throat Chakra deals with all issues relating to self-awareness in personal relationships. During the age of five you become aware of yourself in relation to the people closest to you: your family and friends. You learn how to communicate and express yourself. You become aware of how those closest to you treat you. You notice whether or not they approve of you. Through their attitudes about you, you begin to develop your own attitude about yourself. You develop your sense of self. Your self-esteem takes form. This is the chakra where you establish, 'this is who I am.'

About the Chakra

The Throat Chakra is your center for self-knowledge. This is the chakra where your intelligence and your creativity are developed, where you begin to learn. You become aware of what is right and wrong. Your sense of integrity takes root.

The gland associated with this chakra is the Thyroid gland. This gland controls your metabolism and the way your body uses energy. How you feel about yourself is closely tied in to how this gland operates. If your sense of self is good, your metabolism will be good and your body will use energy effectively. If you think poorly of yourself, you will have problems.

Blocked Energy Manifestations

Any kind of trauma or event occurring during this age will manifest as problems in the following areas:

How you communicate,
How you express yourself whether it is through your
  creativity, intelligence, or any special talents
How you relate to the people closest you
Physical problems with speech or hearing
Self-esteem
Personal integrity
Learning disabilities

Emotions

Emotions dealing with integrity:
  Being good/ being bad
  Being honest/ lying
  Cheating/ being cheated/ being lied to
  Stealing/ being robbed
Jealousy
Approval/ disapproval
Feeling criticized/ criticizing others
Feeling smart/ stupid
Feeling snubbed
Feeling nice/ malicious

Feeling offensive/ offended
Feeling disregarded, like no one is listening to you
Feeling misunderstood

Possible Health Problems from Energy That Has Been Blocked Yoo Long

Thyroid problems
Learning disabilities
Throat problems
Speech problems
Hearing problems
Ear problems
Problems with the larynx, esophagus
Sinus problems
Lower, neck problems
Problems with shoulders, parts of the arm, elbow, wrist and hand[9]

Questions to Ask Yourself

Bring yourself back to the age of five and see if you can remember anything unusual, outstanding, or traumatic that happened to you. Did anything happen to your family, did you move, someone die, get sick, get caught in a violent earth or weather condition, etc? If so, examine how the event affected you in the above areas.

Example: When Arthur was five years old, his mother became ill. His father sent him off to a parochial boarding school with little explanation as to what was going on in the family. When he got to school, he ended up rooming with five other boys, all of whom were troubled and disruptive. When Arthur grew up, he didn't know how to express himself, or confront people. This especially showed itself in the way he lived. Arthur kept selecting roommates who were selfish and disruptive; like the roommates he had when he was in parochial school. He would let people walk all over him. If someone did something bad to him, he wouldn't know how to confront him, to ask why. Arthur hated his father for sending him away without any explanation. It wasn't until Arthur confronted his pain about what his father did that he was able to finally speak up for himself. Once he did, he was able to communicate his needs, and live peacefully with more caring people.

Was this the age you first started going to school?

The first time you were sent off to school will feel like abandonment to the soul, especially if your mother didn't work and stayed at home to care for you. Being stripped of her love and of having her near, will feel like a tremendous loss and will play out later in your life in one of the above areas.

Did something happen to you at school?

If yes, remember what it was. What was the belief system it created in your subconscious? How did it affect you later in life?

Example: When Ellen was five and in kindergarten, she brought a dollar bill to school. She placed it in her cubby for safekeeping. During lunch, she went to retrieve it and noticed it was gone. Defiantly, Tommy the class bully, waved it in her face, showing her he had taken it. He challenged her to get it back. Ellen went to the teacher for help. But Miss White brushed her off and told her to handle it herself. Later in life, Ellen owned her own business. One day, Ellen discovered one of her employees was stealing from her. When she went to the police to prosecute, the police turned her away, telling her she didn't have enough evidence. The incident from kindergarten taught Ellen that it was okay for people to steal from her and get away with it. She would receive no help from those in authority.

If there was a problem in the family, how did your family deal with it?

Was your family verbal and freely talked about the problem? Or were things buried or kept hidden? Look to see if all problems were considered equal. In other words, were physical situations handled in the same way as emotional problems? If there was a big problem, did your family seek outside help? How are you today in handling your problems? Do you follow in your family's footsteps?

If you had a problem, how did your parents respond?

Were your parents supportive? Did they help you? Stand behind you? When you have a problem today, how do people respond to you? Are you able to express yourself? Are you able to tell others about your problems, and ask for help? Or are you silent, waiting for those around you to notice on their own, expecting them to read your mind? When others don't notice that you have a problem, do you feel let down, and rationalize to yourself that if they truly loved you, they would notice? Or do you try to work your problems out on your own, feeling that it is useless to go to others?

Did your parents listen to you?

When you talked to your parents, was their attention focused solely on you? Or did they seem distracted? How good are you at getting people to listen to you today?

Example: A woman and her young daughter came into my bookstore one day to buy an alternative health book for a friend diagnosed with cancer. As the woman began describing her friend to me and what she needed, her daughter began making a fuss. I immediately showed the daughter the toys we kept on hand for such a situation. The daughter began playing with them, but just as the mother began talking again, the daughter immediately ran back and started whining. I knew the mother was in the middle of a learning lesson. I could feel how she was trying to bury her anger. So I immediately asked permission if I could stop her for a second and get her to observe what was taking place. She was open-minded and agreed. Meanwhile, the daughter was still grabbing at her, whining and making a scene. I asked the mother what she was feeling having her daughter behave like this? The mother began by talking about how angry and helpless she felt not having any time for herself. Her daughter was constantly demanding attention. I asked the mother to close her eyes and get in touch with the emotion. I guided her through the process of feeling it. As soon as she started releasing the energy, the daughter immediately quieted, walked back to the toys, sat down and played. I immediately pointed this out to the mother. Then I asked her if she could remember a similar incident happening to her when she was young. The tears began to flow as she remembered. Her mother would sit on the phone so long talking with her friends, she felt neglected. One day while her mother was on the phone, she got so fed up she threw a tantrum. Her mother punished her severely for her actions, and said terrible things to her.

"How old were you when this incident happened?" I asked her.

"I must have been around five," she replied.

"And how old is your daughter now?" I asked.

"Five," she replied.

I then told her to observe her daughter's behavior. The daughter was playing happily with the toys. I then explained how children are sensitive to our energies, that when they act up, they are usually feeling the discordant energy of our own blocked emotions. If she would take a moment to feel her emotions and release them before reacting to her child's tantrum, she would save herself future battles with her daughter.

Were your parents strict or demanding, forcing you to bend to their will?

Were there a lot of rules in your house growing up? Were you allowed to express yourself freely, or did you have to fit the mold your parents thought you should be?

When you didn't follow one of their rules, what was your punishment? Was it physical like a spanking, or being sent to your room? Or was your punishment more emotional? Did they withhold their love? Were they verbally abusive? Or were they the opposite, giving you the 'silent treatment' instead?

If your parents were too oppressive, and made too many demands, how did you compensate? Did you do poorly in school? Did you learn to tune them out by developing hearing problems or learning disabilities? Did you rebel, or try to runaway?

How are you today? Are you still subconsciously following your parent's rules and punishing yourself for not being the way they wanted you to be?

Example: One day a grandmother was telling me that she just discovered that her grandson had learning disabilities. She was very upset, because her son, the father, was doing little to help her grandson. He was too busy working and didn't have time. So I asked her to get in touch with the emotion she was feeling. She said she was feeling like a bad parent. Her son never listened to her. I asked her how her parents were with her when she was a child. She replied that they came from Europe and weren't great parents. They didn't have time to listen to her. They were too busy trying to make a living. That's why, she explained, she went out of her way to talk to her son, and be available for him when he needed her.

We talked further. In the end I showed her how in all four cases the emotion was the same, that it had passed down through four generations until it finally became a physical problem. Her parents didn't talk or listen to her. She didn't feel those emotions. Instead she acted them out by polarizing them: she talked too much to her son. He felt she was too smothering and stopped listening. Unfortunately, he stopped listening to his son, too. His son, her grandson, snowballed the emotion into a physical disability by not being able to hear things correctly. By having a learning disability, the grandson learned a way in which he could receive extra attention.

Was one of your parents overbearing? This could be in voice, attitude or in physical presence.

Did one of your parents scare you with their size, their demeanor, or their loud booming voice? Did you feel threatened whenever you were allowed to speak? If you stutter today, or have speech problems, look back to your childhood and see if you felt threatened in any way.

Did one of your parents command attention at your expense?

Did one of your parents have to be the center of attention? At family gatherings, who was is in control? Did you ever feel it was at your expense? Were you frightened to speak up? Were you ever put on the spot, feel shamed or stupid? Or the opposite, never noticed, and felt neglected?

Who is in control today? Do you find that you have taken on your parent's role because that is what you were taught? Or do you polarize what they did by doing the opposite, because what you remember is too painful?

Were you allowed to have your own opinion?

Were you allowed total freedom to have your own opinion or were conditions placed on it? Did your opinion have to be logical to be accepted, scientific, non-emotional, creative, expressed quietly, or with other certain conditions? Were you laughed at or rejected if you didn't comply?

How did your parents feel about your intelligence?

Did you feel smart enough? Or too smart? Did rivalry exist between you and other siblings over who did better in school? Did you feel you were loved better or worse because of your intelligence? What was your family's belief system around education? Were they prejudiced thinking that men are smarter than women; that a woman's place is in the home etc.?

How has this affected how you use your intelligence today? Were you made to feel stupid so you are always signing up for new classes, trying to learn something new, reading a lot of non-fiction, always trying to improve yourself, keeping yourself current with world events?

Did your parents pressure you into studying, being smarter?

Did your parents make you feel stupid, that you are not good enough? Do you have problems today with low self-esteem? Do you have to try harder? Do you feel that the tasks you undertake are overwhelming?

How did your family treat each other?

Were you taught to respect each other? Or were you taught that it was permissible to emotionally abuse each other, or make fun of each other?

Were you made to feel that only 'blood' could be trusted, that 'outsiders' could never be like family? Do you find in your relationship today with your mate and his family, that there is a part of you that mistrusts them because they are not 'of your blood'? Or are you feeling left out for the same reason?

Was one family member pitted against another? Were hidden agendas played out to create hate and animosity among each other?

Example: Tom grew up with two other brothers, who were close in age. Their father set tough standards. His approval was hard to come by. Tom and his brothers became very competitive over who could get that approval. They tried different ways of sabotaging each other to make themselves look better. When Tom grew up and started to work, he had difficulty keeping a job. His bosses all complained about the same thing: that Tom didn't know how to get along with his associates. He didn't know how to be a team player.

How much criticism did you receive?

If you are having thyroid problems today, then I can tell you that you received too much criticism. If criticizing each other was a normal family occurrence, then you learned how to dish it out and receive it.

Think of criticism in terms of energy. Imagine that you are being criticized every day. Think of each time you are being criticized as a spear of negative energy being shot at you. Where do you think that energy goes when it hits you? If you are not dissipating the energy by feeling the emotional hurt, then that energy gets stored in your body. Your thyroid gland is where that particular energy gets stored.

Were you seeking approval and not getting it?

Do you feel that your parents approved of you? How did they show you they approved? Did they verbally tell you, physically demonstrate it, tell others so you heard it indirectly? How do you receive approval today?

If you didn't get the approval you needed as a child, how is that reflecting in your life today? Are you attracting people who are like your parents, who still don't approve of you?

Do people misunderstand the things you say or do?

Do you go out of your way to help people, only to have it backfire on you in the end? Or do you say things that people take the wrong way? If yes, go back to your childhood and see if there is a particular event in which you felt misunderstood.

Did anyone put you down, making you feel bad about yourself?

Did anyone in your family or your friends ever tease you or put you down, making you feel bad about yourself? This could be about how you looked, acted, spoke, etc. Are you still carrying scars? Are you going out of your way today not to be like the way you were so you don't get teased again? For example, were you teased for being fat, and now you are determined to stay thin? Were you teased for having funny teeth, which makes you careful how you smile today? Were you teased for the way you look, which made you undergo plastic surgery? If you didn't first deal with the buried hurt, no matter how much you change your physical condition, you will still not feel good about yourself.

How was the morality in the family? How were you treated if you lied, stole, etc.?

If you came from a morally upright family, what was your punishment if you were bad? Are you still punishing yourself that way today?

Was the moral atmosphere so strict that today you set such stiff rules to live by that you have little fun? Or was the condition just the opposite? The moral fiber in your family was so weak, you go out of your way today not be like them? If yes, what is your greatest fear in being like them?

How did your parents encourage your creativity or special talents?

Were you taught to express them freely; taught they had value? Or were you taught to stifle them or sabotage them?

If you use your creative talents today in your work, how is your work received? Are you successful and prosperous? If not and you are struggling, go back to the age of five and remember your parent's attitudes towards you. Also, remember your parent's attitude about work. Did they tell you that you wouldn't be able to support yourself singing, painting, writing, or being creative?

10

The Moon Center Chakra Zone 6 (Color: Orange)

Developmental Age

The Moon Center Chakra develops during the age of six.

Developmental Theme

The Moon Center Chakra deals with issues relating to self-awareness in society. At the age of five, a child learns how to relate to his family and those closest to him. At the age of six he looks beyond his home to the outside world where he learns to relate to strangers, and society. Observing others, he begins to compare himself. As he compares himself, he establishes a criterion of self-judgment, of how he measures up. Therefore, self-esteem, which began to develop in the Throat Chakra, also develops in this chakra, yet on a much broader level.

The Moon Center Chakra deals with how you function in society; how you follow society's rules, your morals, how you judge yourself and others, how you fit in, and what are your duties and responsibilities. This is also the time when sexual orientation becomes noticeable. If you are homosexual, the age of six is when you will first begin to notice that you are different. The hypothalamus gland is associated with this chakra, and one of the functions of this gland deals with the sex drive. Recently scientists discovered that this gland is enlarged in males who are gay.

About the Chakra

There is very little information written about the Moon Center Chakra. Yet I consider this chakra to be one of our most important. The Moon Center Chakra invokes life. Within the chakra lies the medulla oblongata, and found within the medulla oblongata are the life sustaining centers which command the heart to beat and the lungs to breathe. Also within this chakra lies the hypothalamus gland. This gland is considered the master gland in the body, because it relays messages from the body to the pituitary gland, and tells the pituitary which hormones the body needs.

In Eastern religions, this chakra is considered a minor chakra. But through my own spiritual experiences, I discovered the Moon Center Chakra to be one of our most important. Because of what I discovered, I can't help feeling that Eastern gurus and enlightened masters deliberately kept this chakra a mystery because of its power. I say this because I believe that unblocking and clearing the energy from this chakra is one of the last things you do before you become enlightened. In Eastern philosophies, enlightenment is a state of bliss achieved through divine realization. This is when you feel you are one with God and have attained everything. Buddha, Jesus, Elijah, Moses, and Mohamed are just a few of the spiritual masters that have attained enlightenment.

A more modern definition of enlightenment concerns the brain. I believe you become enlightened when you know how to use one hundred percent of your brain. Most people use only a small portion of their brain. I believe the Moon Center Chakra is instrumental in activating the parts of the brain we rarely use. These parts of the brain deal with knowing and understanding subtler, subatomic energy.

The highest state achieved in meditation is transcendence. Transcendence is no different than being in the deepest state of sleep—Delta. Delta is the state when the body is in its healing mode, when feelings of well being are experienced. Scientists have discovered that the low, back portion of the brain is activated during Delta. This part of the brain is associated with the Moon Center Chakra.

Through my spiritual experiences, I discovered that the Moon Center Chakra is the doorway to knowing subtler subatomic energies. In other words, it is the doorway to other worlds, where spirit is accessed. How many times have you felt the hairs rise at the back of your neck when you sensed a ghost or spirit present? How many times have you felt goose bumps run down your skin when you heard something that rang with spiritual truth? The spirit world sits in the same space you do, only its atoms are vibrating at a different frequency so you can't see it. The Moon Center Chakra helps you to access it.

Whenever spirit communicates to me, I feel it as a burst of love from within me and a flowing wash of love outside me. Sometimes my skin tingles or rises with goose bumps. Whenever spirit communicates to me, I feel it simultaneously in two places, outside me and inside me. I call this a feeling of grace. In the beginning, in feeling the love outside me and inside me, I became aware of how I exist on different levels, all at the same time. I became aware that I am spirit, or energy, at the same time I am human, and that both are in constant communication.

When I think of the Moon Center Chakra, once again, the Bible's tale of Adam and Eve comes to mind. I find the story of the Garden of Eden rich in symbolism. When Adam and Eve took a bite out of the apple, and were thrown out of the Garden of Eden, the first emotion they felt was shame. They felt shame about their nudity and what they did.

Shame is the first emotion we feel when we enter the body. As spirit, before the soul takes over and reduces our energy, we are in a state of total love, where we are empowered, where we have everything we want, where we know we are one with God. But after the soul reduces our energy so we can fit into a body, we are literally stripped of everything. We suddenly find ourselves as helpless little babies and powerless to the whims of our parents. When this happens, the overriding emotion we feel is shame. Shame sits deep in the soul. When the soul commands life to begin, it begins in the Moon Center Chakra, where our first breath is sparked by the medulla oblongata. The Moon Center Chakra then becomes the repository where shame sits.

In my experiences in working with people, I found shame to be one of the hardest emotions to feel. Yet shame is one of the most powerful and important of the emotions. Shame teaches us how to communicate with our spirit. It teaches us how to begin to connect to the spirit world, to God. In other words, shame teaches us how to get back to the Garden of Eden. It does this by making us aware that we have an energy field surrounding us. All the other emotions we feel, we feel inside our bodies. Yet when we feel shame, we not only feel it inside our bodies, but outside our bodies as well. Next time you feel shame, notice how it feels different than the other emotions. Notice how on in the inside you feel like you are being crushed by the emotion, while at the same time on the outside, your skin is burning with it. Being able to feel energy simultaneously in both places is the beginning process to feeling the bigger you—you, and your spirit.

Therefore, the emotions found in the Moon Center Chakra teach us to become aware of our energy fields. By becoming aware of our energy field we then learn how to communicate with spirit and know energy. By communicating with spirit, we tap into our intuition, our soul's desires, and to God. We also tap into the energy fields of those around us, alive and dead. The Moon Center Chakra is our doorway to this subatomic world.

To have easy access to the subatomic world, our energy fields must be free of emotional blocks. Self-judgment and guilt, therefore, become key issues in this chakra. Each time we judge ourselves or feel guilty, we stop the process of allowing an emotion to be expressed. Each time we stop an emotion from being expressed, we stop the flow of energy in the body. This creates a block in one of the chakras.

Each energy block, every emotion we don't feel, is a closed door blocking our entrance into the spirit world. As we unblock the energy and feel those emotions, we open the doors, allowing greater access to the spirit world. As we open more of those doors, communicating with spirit gets easier. The Moon Center Chakra keeps track of all the blocks in the other chakras. It is not much different than the hypothalamus gland, which keeps track of the body, then tells the pituitary what the body needs. The Moon Center Chakra does the same thing. It keeps tabs of the energy blocks in the body, then relays the information to the soul.

Besides being a conduit to the world of energy and spirit, the Moon Center Chakra is also a passageway for the soul. Through my years of spiritual study, I experienced this several times. The first time occurred when I had an out of body experience and witnessed everything as pulsating energy. I relate this experience in the introduction of this book. Other times I saw the soul detach itself from inside the body and sit on the back of the neck at the Moon Center Chakra. I witnessed it in people who were seriously ill and getting ready to die. And once I witnessed it with my son while he was playing volleyball. His soul was thrown out of his body, through his Moon Center Chakra, when another player rammed him in the chest. As his soul sat on the back of his neck, I watched my son stagger to the ground, be disoriented and throw up. It wasn't until a few minutes later when his soul returned to its proper location in his chest, that my son felt fine again as though nothing happened.

In viewing auras, people who pray a lot have a bright white light glowing from their Moon Center Chakras. These people have developed a strong communication link with God, even though they might not realize it.

People who channel have this strong link too. The Moon Center Chakra is used to relay information from the spirit world. When I channel, the back of my neck becomes stiff as I feel spirit sending me messages to pass on to others.

Besides being the doorway to the spiritual world, the Moon Center Chakra is also concerned with the physical world and how you feel about it. People who have strong morals, who are concerned with being good or bad, are people with Moon Center Chakra issues. These are people who feel very connected to society and in following society's rules.

Also responsibility is a key issue of The Moon Center Chakra. I am going to define responsibility as being morally accountable for an action. In other words, it is doing something because you have to, or because it is expected of you, not because you want to. In my estimation, self-judgment and responsibility go hand in hand. Remember what I stated previously about self-judgment. Self-judgment creates the blocks that keep you from knowing your energy field and the sprit world. I call self-judgment the past tense of responsibility. When you are judging yourself, you are thinking about something that happened in the past. You are analyzing it because you are unhappy about the outcome. You are saying to yourself, "I *should have* done it this way, not that way." Instead of feeling the emotion that caused you to act that way, you are instead rationalizing how you acted: you are making excuses, justifying your actions, blaming others, thinking about how you will act differently next time, etc, etc.

Responsibility is self-judgment in the present tense. When you are being responsible, you are saying to yourself, "I *should* do this." Instead of tuning into the emotion that is causing you to be responsible, you are forcing yourself to *think* about your commitments, and what must be done. Both self-judgement and responsibility keep you in a thinking mode and guard you from feeling an emotion. I find that people who think too much at the expense of feeling their emotions usually end up paralyzed, or off their feet.

All movement comes to halt. Emotion moves energy. Without emotion, there is no movement.

The Moon Center Chakra is where life and death is decided. This is the chakra that houses the life sustaining centers found in the medulla oblongata. The first breath of the body is activated in this chakra, so is the last breath. If there are too many emotional blocks that bar contact with spirit, then spirit may decide to forgo the body. In other words, death occurs. Also, the feeling of wanting to kill yourself is an emotion found in this chakra. If you are suicidal, look back to the age of six to see if you experienced any traumas that caused you to feel this way.

Blocked Energy Manifestations

Life lessons will deal with any type of self-judgment, guilt, self-esteem, feeling different, or issues relating to wanting to live or die. Also, people who have experienced a trauma during this age might feel too responsible, not responsible enough, too moral, immoral, or too hard on themselves and others.

The portion of the spine associated with this chakra is the upper neck. Any traumas that happen during the sixth year life will manifest as problems later with the hypothalamus gland, the lower brain, teeth, bones, skin, hair, joints, muscles, ligaments, and the immune system.

Previously, I wrote that the immune system is part of the Heart Chakra, where the thymus gland is found. Yet time after time, in working with people who suffer with immunity problems, I discovered the source of their problems to be an energy block in the Moon Center Chakra. In researching the immune system, I discovered that the thymus gland begins to degenerate after puberty, and that afterwards, bone marrow becomes the primary source for creating immunity in the body. Since the skeletal system is part of the Moon Center Chakra, this then makes sense why I find energy blocks there. Therefore, the Moon Center Chakra becomes the main energy center for the immune system. I associate the Heart Chakra with the immune system in only a minor way.

Emotions

Self Judgment
Guilt
Feeling responsible/ irresponsible
Shame
Disgust
Humiliation
Embarrassment
Feeling different
Feeling like you don't belong
Feelings of being good or bad
Feeling like you want to die
Feeling not good enough

Possible Health Problems from Energy That Has Been Blocked Too Long

Hypothalamus gland problems
Autism
Paralysis
Teeth, gum problems
Skin or hair problems
Bone, joint, muscle problems
Arthritis
Problems with the immune system
Asthma
Cystic Fibrosis
Emphysema
AIDs
Infections, viruses

Lower brain problems
Upper neck problems
Some shoulder, arm, elbow, wrist or hand problems[10]

Questions to Ask Yourself

At the age of six, were there any traumas in your life?

Did anyone die? Did you move? Did anything happen at school? Were there any unusual weather conditions or catastrophes? Were you in any accidents? Was someone in your family sick or injured? Did you take any trips? Did your parents take any trips without you? How was the financial condition of your family? Was their marriage good? Any type of trauma experienced during this age will affect your self-esteem and how you relate to society. Check the Blocked Energy Manifestation section to see how else you could be affected.

How responsible are you?

Think about your responsibilities. How many do you do because you enjoy doing them? How many do you do because you think you have to? If you are doing them because you *should* or *have* to, then chances are there is a blocked emotion causing you to feel that way. To get in touch with this emotion, think about the responsibility you hate doing. While you are thinking about it, allow your emotions to surface. Follow the System For Soul Memory to feel the emotion and release it.

For example, on his deathbed, Sandy's father made her promise to watch over his new wife after his death. Sandy agreed. For two years, she was diligent in calling her stepmother and making sure everything was fine. Yet Sandy hated making the calls. She put them off as long as she could. She didn't like her stepmother and thought her selfish. One day during a call, Sandy's stepmother told her not to call again. She told Sandy that her calls were making her feel terrible, like she was a burden. Sandy was appalled and felt guilty hearing the truth. She felt like she was betraying her father in not following his deathbed wishes.

In talking to Sandy and getting her to feel her emotions, Sandy realized how much she hated talking to her stepmother. Her stepmother was too caustic and critical. Sandy pushed those feelings aside in order to follow her father's wishes and be the dutiful daughter. Getting Sandy to feel her emotions was difficult because there was so much guilt in the way. But once Sandy did, she remembered an incident when she was six. An out-of-state cousin came to visit for a month. Sandy was forced to relinquish her bedroom, so her cousin could have it. When Sandy complained, her father made her feel guilty for being so selfish.

When something happens how often do you think about it?

When an event occurs, how much time do you spend thinking about it afterwards? If you notice that you are spending a great deal of time, then you have a blocked emotion sitting behind it. Take a moment to see what it is.

Also, notice what you are thinking about. If you spend a great deal of time worrying about one situation, like how you are going to pay the bills, then you have a blocked emotion. The condition of poverty is a blocked emotion.

When an event occurs, do you later spend time thinking how you should have reacted instead?

Every time you find yourself doing this, you are in self-judgment. Instead of wasting time *thinking* about it, take a moment to feel the blocked emotion sitting behind the event. Feeling the emotion is the only way you will be able to change the situation in the future.

How much rationalizing or justifying do you do?

When something happens, do you spend time afterwards trying to understand it and think it through? Naturally you will say yes, for this is a common occurrence. But next time notice if you are doing it at the expense of feeling your emotions. Working with people, I found that those who are smarter than average, have a greater tendency to rationalize and justify. These people rely on their intelligence at the expense of feeling their emotions. Because they do this, they later end up with back problems or situations where they are off their feet for periods of time.

For example, Brian's mother and father were school teachers. They were very bright people and taught Brian early how to be rational and discuss things openly. When Brian was six, his parents got a divorce. The divorce was friendly, and they were open with Brian and weren't afraid to discuss the situation with him. Even to this day they talk about how mature Brian was through the entire ordeal.

When Brian was thirty-nine, he fell off a horse. He became a quadriplegic. He was totally paralyzed, and couldn't breathe. A respirator kept him alive. The first few months of his hospital stay were harrowing. He almost died several times. Brian's wife, Linda, was by his side constantly, encouraging him to be strong.

Before this, Brian was married once, and in several serious relationships that didn't work out. Linda was the first woman Brian felt really good about. She reminded him of his mother. They were married a year when Brian had the accident.

The accident was the first time Brian was confronted with strong emotions he didn't know how to feel. He only knew how to rationalize them. All the emotions that surfaced were the same emotions he rationalized and didn't feel when he was six years old, when his parents got divorced. Everyday he battles for life, yet, emotionally, he feels like giving up and dying. Because of Linda he pushes the feelings aside. Everyday he is told to be strong. Yet in reality he feels overwhelmingly helpless. But he pushes the feeling aside to show everyone how determined he is. Shame surges within him everyday when he is bathed and his most intimate needs are taken care of, but he avoids the emotion, by laughing and joking with the nurses. The doctors told Brian that they didn't think he would get better. As long as Brian avoids feeling his emotions, the doctors will be right.

Do you constantly find yourself in situations where you feel you don't belong?

Is there any part of your life where you feel out of place? If so, think about your childhood and where you learned to feel out of place.

For example, Jeff grew up in a house where he was the only boy of five children. Jeff's father was a doctor and not around much. The women ruled the household. Female activities dominated, and what they wanted overruled anything Jeff wanted to do. Because of this, Jeff never felt like he belonged. When he grew up, Jeff lived in places where he never felt comfortable or felt like he belonged. Why? Because growing up in that type of environment conditioned him to live in that type of atmosphere. Only when Jeff felt the emotions of feeling rejected and invalidated, was he able to break the training.

How often do you compare yourself to others?

Do you watch TV or the movies, read about people in books and magazines, and want to be just like them? Every time you do this, you are telling yourself you are not good enough the way you are. Take a moment and think about which areas you do this most. Once you do, you will be able to discover the blocked emotion sitting behind it.

Do you guard yourself against others?

The next time a stranger approaches you, observe yourself and notice what you do? Do you unconsciously put up an emotional or mental barrier to protect yourself? What type of defense mechanism do you use? Your skin is your body's largest protective surface. If you are having any problems with your skin, notice how you are using it to shield yourself. What is the emotion you are trying to hide?

Do you feel different than the people around you? Do you have some sort of physical condition, talent, handicap, disease, etc. that makes you feel different?

How do you feel different? What is the emotion that is causing you to feel this way? Did something happen at the age of six that made you feel this way?

If you feel different, what do you do about it? Do you go out of your way to exaggerate your difference? Or do you bury your feelings and try to conform?

Were there any traumas, sexual or just humiliating that made you feel ashamed?

The first time you know shame is at the age of six. Even if you have any sexual traumas or embarrassing situations earlier or later in life, you still experience shame at the age of six. The learning lesson of shame will first be introduced during the development of the Moon Center Chakra.

For example, Rosemary can't remember much about her early years, but she does remember being sexually molested as a teenager by a camp counselor. Rosemary kept the incident a secret. She never dealt with her feelings of shame, anger, and helplessness. When Rosemary went to college, she was date raped by a fellow classmate. Once again, Rosemary kept the incident a secret and didn't deal with her emotions. She was too ashamed to tell anyone. Six months later, Rosemary began having trouble with her teeth. When I saw Rosemary, she was married and had a daughter who was six. She was worried about leaving her daughter in day care. When I spoke to Rosemary, she had just come from the dentist, where she was having work done on her mouth. Every time Rosemary spoke to me, she covered her mouth with her hand so I wouldn't see her missing teeth. In talking to Rosemary, I got her to see how she was living the emotion of shame through her teeth instead of feeling it. Once Rosemary felt her shame, her teeth stopped giving her problems.

Is there a certain type of person who disgusts you?

If yes, then something happened when you were six that made you disgusted by that type of individual.

Example: Ann can't understand why Joe, her husband, is so critical of her weight. Joe is always telling her how fat women disgust him. In feeling the disgust, Joe realized how the feeling evolved. He was six and in first grade. One afternoon he was eating lunch in the school cafeteria, when he accidentally spilled his milk all over the floor. The teacher in charge yelled at him for being so careless. She was fat and wasn't happy that she had to clean the mess herself. Joe never forgot the incident. He always hated the teacher for shaming him in front of his friends.

11

The Third Eye Chakra Zone 7 (Color: Yellow)

Developmental Age

The Third Eye Chakra develops during the age of seven.

Developmental Theme

The Third Eye Chakra deals with issues relating to one's beliefs, and what one does with them. At the age of seven children become more aware of their universe. They begin to ask questions. They wonder more about their existence, where they come from, and what is their purpose. Beliefs are established. These beliefs deal with God, religion, science, law, and ethics. Any trauma, which happens during this year, will set the stage for the future in what children do with their beliefs, and how others react to them.

About the Chakra

Your life is a creation of your beliefs. Energy that is stored in the Solar Plexus Chakra is pulled up the shushumna, the nadis-passageway found in the spine, and pulled out the Third Eye Chakra to create the world of your beliefs. If you look at your life at this moment, at the way you live, your relationships to people, to money, your health, etc., you will see what your beliefs are.

The System For Soul Memory believes there are two types of belief systems that operate in the body. The first system operates from *conscious* beliefs. Conscious beliefs are the thoughts you think up and *know* about. They are the ideas you formulate, imagine, and create, and the intentions you set out to accomplish. Conscious beliefs change as often as you want.

The second type of belief system operates from *subconscious* beliefs. Subconscious beliefs are comprised of felt and unfelt emotions, and the seed patterns developed while you experienced them. They produce the daily events of your life and go *unnoticed* like the other autonomic systems in the body until a situation is created that requires them to be noticed. Energy patterns established from subconscious beliefs can only be changed through feeling unresolved emotions.

Found in the Third Eye Chakra is the pituitary gland. The pituitary gland is a link between the central nervous system and the endocrine system. It stores and manufactures the necessary hormones the body needs. It works closely with the other glands of the body to keep the body functioning properly. It is connected to the hypothalamus gland where it receives instructions on which hormones to send to the body.

The Third Eye Chakra operates on an energy level, much the same way as the pituitary gland does on a physical level. It too works closely with the other chakras to keep your life functioning normally, and to create the world of your beliefs. It too is connected to the Moon Center Chakra where it receives information from the soul and the energy fields around you.

Just as the Moon Center Chakra opens the doorway to the subatomic world of energy fields, the Third Eye Chakra allows you to see it. This is the center where intuition and psychic abilities are developed. Also connected to this chakra, is your ability to imagine, daydream, and create and visualize things in your mind.

Being able to visualize is another way to change your future. Visualization is the beginning step to creating. What you see in your mind, you can create, by using the emotions of intent, determination, and will to empower what you see. (Chapter 15 explains in more depth how to manifest.) Therefore, intention, determination and will are important emotions found in this chakra.

The Third Eye Chakra controls the Central Nervous System. Any problems with the central nervous system will relate to issues concerning this chakra.

Blocked Energy Manifestations

Life lessons to be learned through the Third Eye Chakra will deal with issues concerning will, pride, vanity, pretentiousness, self-righteousness, fanaticism, prejudice, persecution, superstition, obsessions, convictions, and religious fervor. Any traumas experienced during the age of seven will manifest in problems in any of these areas.

Emotions

Determination
Pride/ humility
Conceit
Feeling pretentious
Feeling persecuted
Feeling falsely accused
Obsessed
Feeling self-righteous
Feeling brainwashed
Stubbornness
Narrow-minded
Feeling practical, feeling idealistic
Feeling jaded, bored

Possible Health Problems from Energy That Has Been Blocked Too Long

Problems with the Central Nervous System
Pituitary gland problems
Eye problems
Vision problems
Some brain problems caused by injury, stroke or tumors

Questions to Ask Yourself

At the age of seven, did you experience any traumas?

Did you move? Anyone die? Did you experience any accidents or ill health? How was your family life? How was your school life? Did anything unusual happen? If an event occurred that created strong emotions in you, then you will manifest problems in your life in the above areas.

How accepted are your beliefs?

What happens when you give your opinion to others? Is it accepted, rejected, or scorned? If you have a problem having your opinion valued, look back to the age of seven and see if you can remember any traumas that may deal with this.

Example: Arlene has a problem at work. She is feeling unappreciated. Her bosses never comment on the work she does. Yet she knows she is doing a good job. When I asked Arlene what happened at seven, she told me her parents got separated and later divorced. In looking back, Arlene realized that during this time her parents were so caught up in their own problems, they had little time for her. Remembering this helped Arlene feel the old buried emotions. Once she did, she was amazed at what happened. The next day at work, her boss called her into his office to tell her she was doing a good job and that she was getting a raise.

Do you force your will on others? How controlling are you? Or do you allow others to manipulate and control you?

If you use your will or determination to control your life and others, you will eventually pay a price. Exerting your will takes a tremendous amount of energy and can later cause problems in the brain and central nervous system. Anytime you use your will to control others or to control your environment, you are running from a buried emotion you do not wish to deal with. Eventually, the soul will take drastic actions to overtake your will. Take a step back and notice which areas in your life you try to control.

Example: Karen is a professional golfer. She became proficient at golf at a very young age because her home life was miserable. Her parents were always fighting, her mother blaming her father for their misery. To escape, Karen concentrated on golf. Through strong determination, she was able to become a pro. Yet as a pro, she had difficulty making enough money to stay on the tour. Her game especially suffered every time her father visited her on the circuit. It wasn't until Karen faced her father and the old buried emotions that she was able to play better and make more money.

If you allow others to control you, ask yourself why? What happened in your childhood that taught you to give up your free will, or not to exert it?

Example: Julie came to see me for a psychic reading. She explained that she was in a state of limbo, and wanted to know her future possibilities. After the reading, Julie complained that everyone in her family was mentioned except for herself. Nothing was mentioned about her own future possibilities. She wanted to know why. So I explained to Julie that this frequently occurs in people who don't exert their energy and will. Their reading will reflect it. So I asked Julie what happened when she was younger that caused her to bend to the wishes of others and keep her from using her will. This is what she remembered.

When Julie was seven, she convinced her friend Margie to ride their bikes to the local convenience store to buy candy, even though it was against their parents' orders. On the way, Margie was hit by a car and rushed to the hospital. She stayed there for three months. Julie never forgave herself. If she hadn't forced her will on Margie, she never would have been hurt. From that day on, Julie allowed others to guide her. Today, her life was reflecting it.

Do you allow yourself to daydream?

Your soul talks to you through your daydreams. Therefore, notice what you daydream about. Notice the subject matter and try to determine what your soul is trying to tell you. Also, daydreaming is a good tool to develop your creativity, and hone your visualizing skills.

How do you accept your creativity?

What are your feelings about your creativity? Are you creative? Do you allow your creative expression free reign, or do you push it aside to operate more logically? How was creativity handled in your family? Was it encouraged, or ignored? Were physical activities like sports, or mental pursuits like learning, considered more important?

If you feel you are not creative enough today, go back to your childhood and examine where you were taught to bury your creativity. If you feel you are creative, but your creative talents are not well received, go back and look for the reason why.

Do you feel persecuted, whether it is through religion, race, or color?

If you are feeling persecuted, look back and notice the attitudes your parents and society taught you. Remember, on the level of the soul, you are asking people to persecute you. What are you subconsciously saying?

Example: Esther is Jewish. Growing up, she was taught that Jews were God's 'Chosen' people. She was also taught how Jews have always been persecuted. She remembered a particular incident happening when she was seven, where a teacher condemned her for missing school because of the Jewish holidays. As she grew older scattered incidents of being persecuted continued to happen. In talking to Esther, and getting her to feel her emotions, Esther realized how she was asking people to persecute her. In believing that she was 'Chosen', she gave herself an air of superiority. In believing that Jews are always persecuted, she subconsciously told people to persecute her. What she had been taught as a child, gave her the belief system that she should be persecuted. Once she realized this, the persecution stopped.

Are your beliefs yours or what others tell you?

Examine your beliefs and see if there are any in which you resist or have trouble with. If you find yourself believing in something, but it is fighting you, or giving you grief, then you must examine the emotions lying underneath. Ask yourself, "Do I really believe this?" Was there something that happened when you were younger that concerned this? Or did you have a personal experience that proved this belief to be false, even though you still hold strongly to the belief?

Do you have a fear of being brainwashed, or hypnotized?

If yes, then look back to your childhood and find where this fear first originated. Did something happen when you were seven that triggered it? Also, don't discount the things you did that weren't traumatic. Did you see a movie or TV program that frightened you? Did you play a game that touched a hidden fear?

How do you feel about your intuition?

Your intuition is your soul talking to you. Are you aware of it? How do you accept it? Do you listen to it. Or do you disregard it? Do you fear it? Or do you bury it because religion told you that it is dangerous, or evil? Maybe you think you don't have it because you haven't experienced it.

Everyone is intuitive. What you do with your intuition now is because of what you were taught when you were young. Your intuition is always telling you things, no matter how much you try to suppress it, or ignore it. If you wish to be more intuitive, all you have to do is tell the soul, and the soul will do the rest. The soul wants you to be more intuitive. If there are any past traumas that keep you from being intuitive, the soul will create them in your life for you to heal. All you have to do is pay attention, and make sure you feel your emotions. The more you feel, the more intuitive you will become.

How easily do you accept changes in your life? How rooted are you to your beliefs?

Every time the soul gains wisdom, beliefs change. In other words, every time you feel an emotion, you are changing your belief system. You are changing the energy system of your body; therefore, you are changing your life. If you can adapt easily to these changes, then you are a person who has a lot of energy movement in your life. You are a person who is not afraid to feel.

12

The Crown Chakra Zone 8 (Color: White)

Development Age

The Crown Chakra develops during the age of eight.

Developmental Theme

The Crown Chakra deals with issues relating to self-truth. Self-truth means knowing yourself, and being in total acceptance of the way you are. In other words, recognizing, accepting and loving all your emotions, actions and thoughts, how you are, who you are, who you were, what you look like, and what you do.

About the Chakra

Just as the Moon Center Chakra is the doorway to the spiritual world, and the Third Eye Chakra allows you to see and hear it, the Crown Chakra allows you to be one with it. Through the Crown Chakra, you are able to experience states of rapture and bliss, to experience love beyond the normal human understanding. Through the Crown Chakra, you learn you are more than your physical body. This chakra enables you to merge and be one with others, to know that you are not really separate. It allows you to experience what a highly powered microscope shows physicists: that everything is comprised of energy and that on the subatomic level, all energy is connected. I call the Crown Chakra the God Chakra, because through this chakra you learn that all energy is God, and that all energy lives: it thinks and feels just as you do.

When all the chakras in the body are free of energy blocks and the Crown Chakra is fully opened, enlightenment occurs. One hundred percent of the brain is fully activated. When you become enlightened, you allow yourself to feel all your emotions. You love and accept yourself just the way you are. When enlightenment occurs, you realize that this is the way God wanted you, and that you are perfect, even with all your imperfections. These emotions lead to feelings of love and a reverence for everything in the universe. You begin to realize that you are one with everything. You have full use of all your psychic abilities. Your telepathic abilities put you in the shoes of others. You know everyone's emotions and thoughts. You experience what they experience, and you love them, recognizing them as being an aspect of God, and also, an aspect of you. There is no difference. No longer is there the feeling of separation you experienced at birth. You remember how it was when you were in spirit. You remember everything that is recorded in your soul. You know everything you wish to know, because you are in direct communication with spirit, and with God. Once you love and accept everything about you, you love and accept everything in others.

The pineal gland, found in the center of the brain, is located in this chakra. Science knows little about this gland. They know it shrinks around the age of puberty, and they believe it affects our sleep cycles, our cirdadian rhythms, our biological clocks and the aging process. The pineal gland produces the hormone melatonin, which science is just discovering helps to ease insomnia, fatigue, and depression.

At the age of eight, children begin to realize their beliefs don't account for much. At this stage in their life, they are living their lives by others standards; how their parents want them to be, how religion wants them to be, and how society wants them to be. They turn away from knowing the truth about themselves. Instead, they look to others to tell them what their truth is.

Interestingly, it is around this time when the pineal gland stops developing and begins its slow decline. I believe there is a direct correlation. Scientists suspect that the pineal gland is affected by endogenous messages such as emotions. When you look outside yourself, it is hard to know what your emotions are and to feel them. It is my belief that once you begin looking inward again, and fully feel your emotions, you begin triggering the necessary responses to restore the pineal gland to its original condition. When the pineal gland is functioning at full potential, you experience higher states of consciousness such as bliss, rapture, and ecstasy. Scientists are finding that chemicals produced in the pineal gland indirectly cause psychedelic experiences, and mental states of well-being.

There is a tract that runs from the pineal gland to the hypothalamus gland. It is the hypothalamus gland that instructs the pineal when to produce melatonin. Therefore, the pineal gland, the pituitary gland, and the hypothalamus gland all work closely to keep the body functioning normally. On an energy level, it is no different. The Crown Chakra, the Third Eye Chakra and the Moon Center Chakra also work closely to keep the energy of the body functioning normally. It does this by integrating emotions with thoughts and experiences, and passing the newly gained wisdom to the soul.

Blocked Energy Manifestations

Any kind of trauma or event that happens at the age of eight will reflect in how you are accepted, and how you accept yourself.

Life lessons will deal with forgiveness, being in denial, feeling validated, and issues involving the truth, deception or phoniness.

Emotions

Reverence
Bliss/ rapture
Feeling accepted
Feeling validated
Feeling like a phony
Feeling forgiveness
Feeling doubt

Possible Health Problems from Energy That Has Been Blocked Too Long

Pineal gland problems
Some problems with the brain such as stroke, tumors and injury
Mental problems
Depression
Alzheimer's Disease
Dementia
Epilepsy
Seasonal Defective Disorder
Sleep problems

Questions to Ask Yourself

At the age of eight, did you experience any traumas or emotional upsets?

Any event that occurred during this age will manifest later as having problems in the above areas.

Are there any emotions you won't allow yourself to feel?

Is there one particular emotion that is so scary you go out of your way not to feel it? Do you know why?

Example: Jay was always afraid of being trapped in a small dark space. Whenever he would read a book or watch a movie where someone was trapped in a small dark space, fear would surge through him. He would immediately stop the feelings of claustrophobia. He couldn't imagine why he felt this way. It wasn't until Jay allowed himself to feel the emotions that he was able to pinpoint the root of his problem. When Jay was eight, he was playing hide and seek with his brother. He was hiding in the closet when his brother decided to play a joke on him, and lock the closet door. Jay remained locked in the tiny dark closet until his mother found him thirty minutes later. Jay always remembered the story, but he never related it to his fear of being trapped. After the realization, Jay never experienced the fear again.

Do you recognize all your thoughts?

Are you aware of what you are thinking? Do you notice that you spend more time thinking about one particular subject more than others? If yes, look to see what blocked emotion is making you think this way.

Also, notice if there are any thoughts you stop and won't allow yourself to think about. Are there any thoughts that create fear in you? Just as with an emotion, fearing a thought means there is still an unresolved issue from the past.

Example: Rick has an aversion to homeless people. He hates looking at them, and thinking about them. Whenever he sees one, he goes out of his way to avoid one. Rick thinks of himself as a caring person. He can't imagine why he has such a strong reaction to homeless people. To understand where his aversion originated, Rick followed the System for Soul Memory and began concentrating on the thought of a homeless person. Rick was surprised at the emotion that surfaced, one of extreme sadness. He allowed himself to feel the emotion, until there was no more emotion to feel. It wasn't until the next day that Rick suddenly knew where his aversion originated. He remembered an incident that happened when he was eight. His family moved to a new home in a different state. On the day of the move, Rick remembered his father abandoning their dog on the side of the highway as they headed out of town. His father wouldn't allow them to take the dog to their new home. Rick felt terrible about abandoning his dog. He knew that once his dog was homeless, he would die. In that moment of clarity, Rick realized how his aversion to homeless people was really a smoke screen hiding his hurt about his dog.

Do you like yourself?

If someone asked you at this precise moment if you liked yourself, what would be your response? If the answer is no, then discover why don't you like yourself. Make a list. For each reason you don't like yourself, you will have a past trauma and a blocked emotion explaining why.

Is there any part of yourself you wish you could change?

Think about what you want to change and why? What do you remember from your childhood that makes you feel this way? Do you want to change because it's your desire or because others want it? Are you doing it to please them?

Example: Andrea is overweight and wants to be thinner. Yet every time she tries losing weight, she fails. Andrea's motivation to lose weight is to feel better. Yet the true motivation comes from her parents. They are thin and health conscious. They tell her that if she doesn't lose the weight she increases her risk of illness.

After Andrea and I spoke, she realized that she was using her weight as a means of getting back at her parents. Subconsciously, she was very angry with them. She never felt like they accepted her. She always had to be better. Andrea was using her weight as a receptacle for her anger. Until she feels her anger and sadness, she will never lose the weight.

How do others feel about you?

How easily do others accept you? If you are not easily accepted, what subconscious signals do you think you send out, telling others not to accept you?

Example: Cecilia always felt left out. Especially after work when her fellow co-workers went out drinking without her. She couldn't figure out why she was never included.

After talking to her and following the System For Soul Memory, Cecilia knew why. She was eight when she was invited to a classmate's birthday party. She was not feeling well; but she was desperate to go, because Ginger was one of the most popular girls in the class, and it was an honor to be invited. She was sitting at the table, eating birthday cake when she suddenly became desperately ill. She threw up all over Ginger's cake and the girl sitting next to her. To this day, Cecilia still remembers the looks of horror and revulsion on the girls' faces. She never resolved the old feelings. Because she still feels disgusted with herself, Cecilia subconsciously tells the people around her to exclude her from their plans.

Growing up, how did your parents feel about you? What messages were they always giving you?

Example: Ever since he could remember, Steve was often told how his parents had to get married because of him. His parent's marriage wasn't a happy one. Steve always felt that his mother blamed him for her unhappy life. After all, if he hadn't come along, she wouldn't have had to get married. Later in Steve's life, this manifested in the way his family and friends accepted him. If you asked Steve, he would be the first to tell you that he was the one always blamed for everything. Like when his best friend's wife had an affair and Steve suspected, but didn't say anything. His friend later blamed him for their divorce. Steve had never connected the way his mother felt about him with his life today. Once he made the connection and felt the buried emotions, people stopped blaming him. His energy field was no longer telling people that he should be blamed.

How easily do you forgive yourself or others?

How hard are you on yourself? Are you the last one to forgive yourself for something you did?

Forgiveness only happens after you have felt all the emotions involved in the situation. You cannot simply say, I forgive. The soul won't let you. The soul demands that you feel your hurt and the hurt you caused another. Many times, guilt or self- judgment gets in the way of allowing you to feel the hurt. In order to understand this better, read Chapter 14.

Do you listen to what others tell you before you listen to yourself?

Are other's opinions more important than yours? People can sense subconsciously if this is the case. A good mirror is to notice when you are in a group of people. Do people value your opinion over others? If you don't rate your opinion highly, no one will. Notice if there is one particular situation where this happens more frequently. For example, does it happen more at work, at home, with your spouse, your parents, your children, etc.? Where it does happen the most is the place where you feel most vulnerable and powerless.

Example: Karen was working as a teacher in an elementary school when she was fired. Her supervisor claimed she wasn't following school guidelines. Karen claimed the students in her class had special needs and she needed to bend the rules to accommodate them. She felt her opinions on this matter overruled those of the school district. She was in the process of suing the school district to get her job back when she came to me. After putting her through The System for Soul Memory, Karen remembered an incident that occurred when she was a child. Her baby brother was born. He was born with a foot problem that required he wear a special brace when he slept. One day, while her mother was gone and a baby sitter was watching them, Karen removed her brother's brace to get him to stop crying. When her mother came home she punished her severely and told her that it was important that she follow the rules. Karen couldn't get her mother to understand that sometimes it was necessary to break the rules. Today, Karen was using the school board to try to resolve those old buried feelings.

Are you the way you are, because you chose to be that way, or because others want you to be that way?

Every time you deny a part of yourself to please someone else, you are being a phony. I have found that people who do this often will attract people into their lives who will be phonies. At some point these people will deceive you. The soul does this to mirror what you are doing to yourself. Therefore, if you have any deception or phoniness happening to you, look at your life and see where you are not being truthful with yourself.

Example: Darren is gay but he lives his life as though he is straight. He is married and has two children. His sex life is almost non-existent, and his wife complains; but Darren tells her he's so stressed from his work as a lawyer that he doesn't have the energy to do both. Darren feels like a phony, especially every time he sees his brother-in-law and feels more attracted to him than his wife. But he loves his children and has no plans of "coming out of the closet."

Darren has a reoccurring problem at work. He has a high percentage of clients who don't pay their bills. It wasn't until after we spoke that Darren realized the connection between his marriage and his work. He saw how because he was feeling guilty about not being straight with his wife, he was punishing himself at work by not having his customers be straight with him.

Are you living the life you were meant to live?

Look back over your life at the opportunities that have come your way. How many of those did you accept? How many did you turn down because it seemed irrational, or you couldn't afford it, or it took you away from your responsibilities?

Example: Gregory was a beautiful child. People would constantly stop him and his mother on the street to tell them. One day, the owner of a talent agency spotted them and gave them his card. He told them that if they were interested in having Gregory work in commercials they should give him a call. Gregory took up the offer and made a nice income doing commercials on a part-time basis. Gregory joined the Screen Actor's Guild, which helped him find even more work. When Gregory graduated from college, he didn't know what he wanted to do. He loved being an actor, but he felt it was too risky a profession to pursue. So even though throughout his life acting jobs kept falling at his feet, Gregory turned his back on acting and became a stockbroker. He wasn't happy doing it, but at least the income was steady. Having a steady income was more important than taking risks and doing what brought him joy.

How often do you doubt yourself or what you do?

Who made you doubt yourself? Look back at your childhood. Was there someone who made you feel unsure about yourself? Did someone say something that later gave you a feeling of inferiority or insecurity? Every time you doubt yourself, you believe the person who doubted you. You are telling yourself, they know more about you than you know.

Example: Charlotte remembers that learning to ride a bicycle was a painful experience. She was terrified of falling and getting hurt, which made her very timid. This exasperated her father, who throughout the ordeal, told her that she was a wimp and would get nowhere in life with that kind of attitude. Charlotte never learned to ride.

This trauma manifested later in Charlotte's life as a fear of driving. Charlotte was so terrified of driving, she waited for someone to drive her where she needed to go. It wasn't until we talked that Charlotte realized she was proving her father's belief true. Because she still believed that she was a wimp, she was creating the reality of 'getting nowhere.'

Do you feel that you are living the genuine you?

Example: Arthur was a daydreamer as a child. He loved to dream up stories, and get lost in his thoughts. Especially in class. Because of this, he was not a good student. His teacher always complained that he could do better if he paid more attention. Arthur remembered one particular incident when he was eight. His teacher caught him daydreaming and decided to make an example of him. He sat him on a stool in front of the class and told the class to keep their eyes on him and not allow him to daydream again. The incident was humiliating for Arthur. So humiliating, that to this day, Arthur guards himself against daydreaming, even though it is still a part of who he is. He works as a cook in a busy diner, at a job that demands he stay focused all the time. He denies himself the joy of dreaming up stories, and chooses to be more responsible instead. He never allowed the genuine him to emerge; nor did he discover what opportunities he missed by do so.

Through my work, I discovered that people who allow themselves to be who they really are and live it, are the people who are the happiest and have the most success in life.

Take the example of Chris. As a child, Chris loved computers. He spent hours playing different computer games. Everything about the computer came naturally to him. When Chris went to college, he never thought to major in what he considered his hobby. He chose a business degree instead. It wasn't until he started doing poorly in his classes, that Chris realized he had a problem. He knew business wasn't the right major for him. His parents told him to switch his major to computers, but the campus counselor told him his grades were so poor, and the computer classes so difficult, that if he did switch he would never graduate. Chris took a semester off and struggled with the situation. He spent the time feeling his emotions. When he returned to college, he returned as a computer major. It took him an extra couple of years to graduate, but when he did, he immediately found a good job working for a large computer company that allowed him to do what he loved doing. Today, Chris is very happy and successful.

13

How to Feel Your Emotions

In working with clients, what struck me most, was how so many of the people I worked with didn't know how to feel their emotions. This chapter will show you how to feel an emotion, and how to feel it in a manner that will satisfy the requirements of the soul.

Emotions are energy. Every time you feel an emotion, you are increasing the level of energy in your body; particularly, if you are feeling an emotion that has long been buried. In which case, you are unclogging the nadis and increasing your life force, allowing your body to hold more energy. In holding more energy, your body begins to change. You become healthier, happier. You open new channels in the brain. Not only do these channels deal with emotions, they deal with reading and understanding energy. These parts of the brain allow you to become telepathic, to read the energy fields of your environment, of others, and to know the energy you are attracting into your life. Some people call these abilities being psychic. I call them instinct. The animals I speak to use these abilities all the time. God gave us these abilities to ensure our survival. Unfortunately, we are trained from birth not to utilize them. Yet, I discovered that people who are raised in abusive or chaotic homes, or anywhere where survival is tough, have honed these abilities and use them frequently.

To be able to feel your emotions, you must change your level of awareness. You must accept that your emotions exist and be willing to look for them. You must be willing to observe them and feel them. This means that every time an incident occurs that upsets you, you must be willing to ask yourself, "What am I feeling?" In working with people who aren't accustomed to feeling their emotions, I noticed, in the beginning, this was difficult to do.

Centering your attention on your emotions, is no different than centering your attention on a particular muscle while doing exercises. In other words, you are focused inwardly: on what is going on inside you, on how it feels both physically and emotionally. It takes practice to train your concentration to do this. Normally all your attention is centered outwardly, on the incident you are involved in and how you are going to respond. Splitting your attention to being aware of what is going on inside you, at the same time to what is going on outside you takes concentrated effort and practice.

In the beginning, as you become accustomed to centering your attention on your emotions, you begin to feel energy as though it was physical. You learn that not all energy feels the same. Some energy feels heavy, some hard, some soft, some good, some bad. As you practice more, and understand energy better, you begin to feel energy take on a more emotional feel. This happens when you begin activating more areas in the brain that allow you to feel energy's subtle variations.

For example, when you first begin centering your attention on your emotions, and you meet someone for the first time, you may only notice that you don't like that person. As you progress, you begin to feel more. The next time you see that person you will know why you don't like him. His energy will feel negative and blocked. After that, as you develop more of your emotional skills, you begin to know why his energy feels bad. You may feel his physical ailments, or the emotions causing them.

As you continue feeling your emotions, and the channels in your brain develop even more, you begin to understand that energy carries information. The brain has the ability to process this information. You already know the brain does this with the cells and molecules inside your body. Your brain also does this with the subatomic energy outside your body. Your brain has the ability to process information from all energy, whether it comes in the grosser form of molecules and cells, or whether it comes in the subtler form of subatomic particles.

You will know you have developed that part of the brain, when the next time you see that person, you receive images of the incident that caused him to be that way, or even perhaps, images of a future event he is getting ready to attract.

As you fine-tune your own sense of awareness and allow yourself to feel even more, you begin to feel even finer, subtler energies. These are the energies of those in spirit, like dead relatives, guardian angels or spiritual teachers. Some people have complained to me that contacting those in spirit is against their religious beliefs, or that it is a bad idea since they could attract negative spirits. This is all a matter of perspective and I always tell people to do what feels best for them. I believe there are several good reasons why you would want to contact them. For myself, I learned that everything is a mirror of me. Like energy attracts like energy. If I attracted a negative spirit into my life, then I am looking at something within me that needs healing. In other words, my soul attracted this negative entity because I had a blocked emotion that needed to be felt. Once I felt the emotion, the spirit was gone. This would be no different than attracting a robber, a rapist, or a murderer into your life. Remember, the soul will do whatever it must to get you to feel an emotion.

Also, contacting spirit allowed me to feel connected to God and all life. It has enriched my life by filling me with incredible love. This love has blessed me with the most incredible experiences and has gotten me through the most difficult times.

In the beginning, the first time you feel an emotion will be very difficult. It will be no different than doing something new, like learning how to use a computer, or learning a difficult dance step. But the more you practice the easier it gets.

Also as you begin to feel an emotion, you will notice that wild, irrational thoughts will surge through you causing you to be anxious and fearful. I call these irrational thoughts, *attachments*. These attachments will cause you to be so fearful and anxious, you will not want to feel the emotion. For example, some of the thoughts I've heard through the years have been: "If I feel this emotion I will die, or be abandoned. I will have nothing and have to live out in the streets. I will kill someone or I will commit suicide. I will go out of control and go crazy and be locked up in an institution, or have a nervous breakdown and be useless, etc., etc." If you logically dissect these thoughts, you will realize how irrational they are. Yet you suffer with them, many times not knowing why you have them or where they come from. Everybody has them. I found them to be part of the natural process of feeling an emotion.

Each emotion in your life has a history. This history begins in your DNA with the history of your ancestors, what they felt and lived. This history also includes all the times the emotion has surfaced in your own life. Every time the emotion surfaced in your life, a different story happened. The subconscious files these stories away by attaching them to the emotion. Unfortunately they get filed haphazardly, so later, when the emotion resurfaces, they come out as being irrational and scary.

For example, the first time Melissa felt abandoned, she was four. Her parents went away on vacation and left her to stay with an aunt who had a large black dog. The dog bit Melissa, making her visit with her aunt a terrifying experience. The next time Melissa felt abandoned, she was a teenager and on a date with her boyfriend. They were at a Friday night high school football game, when her boyfriend became so angry, he ditched her. Melissa had a terrible time finding another ride home. The whole incident was difficult and traumatic. So by the time Melissa was married, and her husband was threatening her with divorce, her irrational, scary attachment to the emotion of abandonment went like this: "If my husband divorces me I will end up homeless. I will be left to die on a dark street, and be eaten by a pack of wild, hungry dogs."

Exercise:

Take a moment to observe the thinking process. I want you to *think* about something. It can be anything, like the last book you read, or the last person you spoke to on the phone, or what you did last weekend. Notice how thinking is a gentle process. The energy is nice, the thoughts come and go easily.

Next take a moment to observe the emotional process. Feel an emotion. To feel an emotion, remember an incident that still bothers you, where the emotion is still raw. Observe what happens when you allow the emotion to surge through you. Notice how the energy of an emotion is different than that of a thought. Notice how it is more powerful. Notice what happens in the body when you feel an emotion. Notice what happens to your thoughts when you allow the emotion to surface.

Emotions are the most powerful spiritual energy you will know. They rise like an explosion through the body. That's why they are feared. They affect different parts of the body. They can make you cry, create mucous, choke you, make you nauseous, make your heart palpitate, make you breathe faster, cause your skin to tingle, to sweat, and to blush. But most especially, emotions make you stop thinking. They don't come from your brain, they come from your body, and as you will learn from this book, your chakras. When strong emotion rules the body, the brain stops to pay attention.

And what does the brain do when this powerful energy erupts? It goes into immediate action to *stop* it. The brain has been programmed to quell the flow of emotional energy. The brain must keep you feeling safe. Remember thoughts feel gentle. That gentle energy feels much safer than the explosive energy of an emotion.

So when an emotion surfaces, the first thing the brain does is to stop it. For a brief second when that emotion surfaced, your awareness was centered on that explosion of energy. As soon as this happened, the brain immediately went into action to bring your awareness back to your thoughts. It quelled the emotion and got you thinking again. Thoughts are safer. With thoughts you can rationalize what just happened. You can figure it out, defend yourself, create safety, protect yourself by thinking, "I shouldn't do that again, or next time I should do this and this so I don't create that surge of emotional energy again." We have given the brain the job to protect us and keep us safe.

When you rationalize, feel guilty, judge yourself, or blame others, you cannot possibly feel an emotion. Your awareness is centered on your thoughts. Anytime your awareness is centered on your thoughts, you cannot feel an emotion. To feel an emotion your awareness must be centered in your body, on your chakras.

Therefore, to feel an emotion, you must stop thinking. You must concentrate solely on the emotion that is taking place. You must move your center of awareness from the brain to the chakra where the energy is being released.

This takes practice. You are so accustomed to stopping the flow of emotional energy and having your brain take charge, that it will take concentrated effort to focus on your emotions rather that on your thoughts. So don't get upset with yourself when you notice you are having trouble doing this. Just accept the fact that this time you stopped the emotional flow but next time you will pay more attention and allow yourself to feel more. If you flag the brain with this command, the brain will comply and allow you to feel more.

The Stages of Feeling an Emotion

In working with people and in observing myself, I have to come learn that there are definite stages to working through an emotion. The stages are as follows:

1. **Fear**
2. **Awareness**
3. **Anger**
4. **Feeling**
5. **Realization**
6. **Release**
7. **Confusion.**
8. **Vulnerability**
9. **Acceptance**
10. **Self-empowerment**
11. **Self trust**

Fear. If you come to think of emotion in terms of energy, it will be easier to understand the process of how an emotion is felt. I found fear to always be the first stage of an emotion getting ready to surface. Fear is the soul's way of telling you that your energy field is getting ready to expand. Because that is exactly what you are getting ready to do. You are going to unclog a nadis, create a better flow of energy through your body and change your life. Many people don't like making changes because it makes them too uncomfortable. This feeling of being uncomfortable comes from the changes taking place in your energy field.

Fear is also created when the emotional attachments surface. Remember, an emotional attachment is the haphazard composition of memories of prior times when the emotion previously surfaced. As soon as fear arises, the brain kicks in and thinks, "Uh oh, I'm going to be in pain again!" This is usually the time when the brain goes into overdrive to quell the emotion and to stop the fear. If you are good at controlling your thoughts and burying your emotions, this will be the time when the emotion is laid to rest. Not until the future, when the soul creates another event to get the emotion to surface again will you experience it. But remember what happens every time you do this. You create an even greater block of energy. Therefore, in the future, the soul must take greater action to free that blocked energy.

Walking through the fear will not be easy. Ask yourself, "What is my biggest fear if I allow myself to feel this emotion?" Many times you will notice that your biggest fear will be the most irrational, or least logical. Or most amazingly, that you have already been living your biggest fear and didn't realize it.

For example, Tina was unhappy in her marriage and wanted a divorce, but was too afraid to go through with it. When I asked her what her biggest fear was, she told me she was afraid of being alone. So I continued to ask Tina more questions. I asked her how much time did her husband spend with her, and how much emotional support did he give her. When we got through talking, Tina realized that her husband paid little attention to her, and that she was already living 'alone.' She was living her biggest fear and didn't realize it! Being in denial and not feeling the emotion of loneliness was triggering Tina's desire for a divorce.

At that point I told Tina what she could expect. If she felt her loneliness, she would change her marriage, and how her husband treats her. If she didn't feel the emotion and divorced her husband, she would still continue the same pattern, which is to experience the loneliness. In other words, the soul guarantees that if she didn't feel the emotion, she would continue living it until she did. She would continue to repeat the love she knew by attracting another man just like her husband who would pay her little attention.

Another response I have heard quite frequently from people is that if they give into the emotion, instead of fighting it, they would be creating the result of the emotion to exist for the rest of their lives. What these people don't realize, is that they are already living the emotion they are fighting. Emotions dealing with survival, such as feeling like a failure, is an emotion that can cause this type of response. These people feel that once they allow themselves to accept that they are a failure, they will be a failure for the rest of their lives. Or once they give into the feeling of poverty and not continue to fight it, they will be poor the rest of their lives.

If this seems to be the case with you, don't get caught up in the 'thinking game' the brain is creating to keep you from feeling the emotion. Instead know you are dealing with the present, not the future. Remember, *Don't think, feel.* Concentrate only on the fact that at this particular moment in your life, you are feeling like a failure. Remember the pendulum and the rules of energy. For every action, there is an equal reaction. For a pendulum to be in balance it must swing both ways. At one end of the pendulum will be success, the other failure. At this moment in your life, your pendulum is swinging towards failure. If you don't allow yourself to accept and feel the failure, the pendulum stays in this position until you do feel it. You won't know success until you have learned what failure feels like.

Awareness. The next stage after walking through the fear will be the awareness of the emotion triggering the situation in your life. Awareness simply means you can name the emotion you are feeling.

Anger. When you become aware of the emotion, anger will come quickly on its heel. Sometimes the situation will be the reverse. You will feel the anger before you realize the emotion. In either case, anger is the *energy stimulator* that will help you to feel the emotion that is causing the situation. Think of the emotion in terms of blocked energy. This emotion has been sitting in your nadis like a blob of cholesterol would sit in your artery clogging it up. Anger is the added dose of stimulation your energy field needs to get this blob out of the nadis and into your energy field so that it can be 'thinned out' and released when you feel it. I call anger a surface emotion because you will find anger attached to almost every emotion you feel. Chapter 14 talks more about this.

How to Feel Anger

Feeling the anger will be very important to feeling the emotion underneath. To properly feel anger, you cannot move a muscle. You cannot utter a word, nor do one thing that is physical. You must pretend your body is paralyzed. Don't confuse *feeling* anger with *acting out* your anger. Acting out anger means yelling, slamming doors, throwing things, hitting things, etc. When you are acting out anger, you are not feeling a thing. Your brain has taken over to stop you from feeling. Instead it has gotten you to play another game, a game that focuses your concentration on your physical movements instead of on the emotion.

To feel anger you must focus your attention inward to the *energy* of the anger. Focusing your attention inward, would be no different than paying attention to a particular muscle if you were lifting weights or doing exercises. You will be putting all your attention on the anger, the energy of it, observing where it sits in your body, and how it makes you feel. The energy of anger is very powerful, like a volcano exploding. At first, it will feel very scary to allow that much energy to be purely released without movement of any kind. But allow yourself to let it flow through you. Continue to think of it as energy.

Feeling. Once you allow all the energy of the anger to flow through you, the emotion hidden beneath will come to the surface. You will know you are finished feeling the anger when this emotion surfaces full force. The emotion will make you cry, feel sad etc. And you will know exactly what the emotion is. Whether it is betrayal, abandonment, loneliness, etc.

When the emotion surfaces, you must also think of it in terms of energy. Keep the emotion flowing. Don't let the brain try and stop it. You can do this by not allowing yourself to think. Instead keep your attention focused on the emotion and the chakra where that emotion is sitting. Then you proceed to feel the emotion in the same way you felt the anger. Don't think or move a muscle, but concentrate all your attention inwardly.

How to Feel an Emotion

1. Center your attention on the emotion to be felt.
2. Notice in which chakra the emotion is sitting.
3. Think of the emotion in terms of energy. Allow yourself to feel the emotion as much as you can. Imagine the chakra in which it resides. Picture it like a balloon. Fill it up with the emotion you are feeling. Blow it up as much as you can with the hurt and pain you are feeling. Imagine your emotion to be the energy filling and expanding the balloon.
4. Picture a knife. Take the knife and slice open the balloon, your chakra. Allow all the pain to flow out of you, to leave you. The *emotional pain* is *energy* leaving you. Concentrate on pushing out the pain through the opening in the chakra. Keep pushing until there is no more pain to push out.
5. When there is no more pain to push out, you have finished feeling the emotion.

If the emotion you are feeling is deeply buried, then you may have to do this procedure several times in order to fully feel the emotion. Remember the image of the clogged artery and imagine your nadis to look the same. It may take several tries to get all the energy unclogged.

Realization. After you have fully felt the emotion, you should remember the seed pattern where that emotion first originated in your childhood. Don't worry if you don't remember the seed pattern. You will still realize past occurrences when that emotion played a role in your life. In the future, you will be able to recognize the emotion easily. It will never be hidden in your subconscious again to create future occurrences.

If a future occurrence does happen again, then the emotion was not fully felt. It is not unusual for another aspect of the emotion to surface and need to be played out. For instance, being abandoned by a parent will feel differently than being abandoned by a friend even though both are the emotion of abandonment. I noticed that if this happens, then one emotion will be the one overriding learning lesson for the person in their life. It is not unusual to have one major emotion be your learning lesson in life. One emotion can have many different aspects and can take lifetimes to explore. In any case, feeling the emotion again will be easier, because once you know how to feel the emotion, you won't be so scared the next time you have to feel it. You will feel more empowered.

Release. After you feel an emotion, there is a tremendous sense of release. This sense of release comes from freeing yourself from all that blocked energy. Also with the release comes a sense of awe. It is spiritually humbling to learn something new about yourself.

Confusion. Don't be surprised if once you feel this release you begin to feel confused. This is the result of your energy field feeling different. It no longer feels comfortable. You are no longer the old you. Your energy field has changed. It has expanded. You are bringing in more energy, and until your body learns what to do with this energy, you will feel confused. Feeling confused may also feel like you are in a void, or a place of emptiness where the new you hasn't yet developed.

Vulnerability. During this time, while you are growing accustomed to your new energy body, you will feel vulnerable. Your old boundaries will no longer exist, and your new ones are not yet familiar. Subconsciously, you won't know where to presence yourself to rebuild your defenses. You won't trust yourself. You will wonder, "If I get myself into the same situation again, how will I handle it?" Give yourself time. It takes time to grow accustomed to your new energy field.

Acceptance. Once you are accustomed to your new energy field, you will notice that your life has changed. The old energy pattern will be gone, replaced by a new one. In the beginning, it will be habit to still look for the old one.

For example, Tina desperately wanted to get married but always seemed to date men who weren't interested in lasting relationships. She always joked with her friends that if they needed a guy who was commitment-shy, they should ask her. She always found them.

Tina was hit hard when she found Martin, fell in love with him, then discovered that her feelings weren't shared. Martin dropped her as soon as he heard Tina wanted marriage. This time Tina finally felt the emotion of rejection. She cried and bemoaned the fact that men always disappointed her. After feeling all the pain, Tina remembered the seed pattern where she first suffered this emotion, and where she developed this pattern. It happened when she was four. Her father promised her he would take her to the Ice Capades, then reneged when an important business meeting took precedence. Her father did this often. He taught Tina early on to expect rejection and to be disappointed.

Two months after Tina had her realization, she was invited on a date by Jerry. Tina really liked Jerry. Because she liked him, Tina waited to be rejected. After all, she was now aware of her subconscious pattern of asking men to reject her. After three months, Tina was still waiting. That's when Jerry told her he wanted to marry her. Tina was surprised. That's when she realized she had changed her energy field and her life by feeling the buried blocked emotions of rejection and disappointment.

Self–empowerment. Not until you are put in a similar situation, and have the chance to re-experience the emotion, will you realize that you won't be so strongly affected by the emotion again. This begins the process of self-empowerment. You realize that you overcame the situation before, and that you can do it again. For instance, later in their relationship, when Jerry broke a date with Tina because he had a business commitment he couldn't avoid, Tina didn't get upset the way she did in the past. Feeling rejected didn't have the same power over her.

Self-trust. When Tina realized this, she also realized that could trust Jerry in a way she could never trust men before. She also realized she could trust herself. She could trust herself to feel her emotions and not be overpowered by them.

Therefore, once you know you can feel an emotion, and you are no longer frightened by it, you gain self-trust. Once you trust yourself, it is easier to feel all your emotions.

Then the true test of knowing you have learned your lesson begins. You know you have learned your lesson when you begin to notice the emotion in others with the same learning lesson. After having experienced it, you begin to feel compassion for them. You begin to feel compassion and love for yourself. You become aware of those people who deal with the emotion, and those who bury it. Those that bury it begin to leave your life. Remember, like energy attracts like energy. You begin attracting new people into your life. Clearly, you see the old patterns, then the new ones, and how you have changed your life.

This happened to Tina. Afterwards, she could spot which friends were having rejection issues. She knew who was going to work it out and who wasn't. Those that didn't became resentful of her, of her new relationship. She felt sorry for them. Eventually they left her life. New friends came in. These friends had strong meaningful relationships. Tina's life changed. Her self-esteem soared and she became happier.

In working with people, I noticed several tendencies concerning how a person feels their emotions. The first has to do with the confusion of *tactile* feeling with *emotional* feeling. When you begin to feel energy, in the beginning, you may feel it as a physical presence instead of as an emotion. For example, if I know someone is having an abandonment issue and I ask him or her to describe what he or she is feeling, if they describe it as a pressure on their chest, then they are sensing the emotion as a tactile feeling instead of as an emotion. Other examples would be feeling agitated, tense, nauseous, a pit in your stomach, all choked up, or having a pain in the body where the emotion sits. You are focusing on the result of what the blocked energy is doing to your body instead of feeling the emotion. If this happens to you, there is an easy way to remedy this. Just continue to stay focused on the tactile feeling. Eventually you will become aware of what the emotion is underneath. Don't be concerned that it may take you a while to discover the emotion. It just means that you are not accustomed to feeling your emotions. It takes time to learn.

Another tendency I noticed, is when I ask people to describe their emotion, they describe their emotion as an action. Instead of feeling rejection, they would say something like, "I feel like he is stabbing me in the heart." Or if they are feeling abandoned, "I feel like running away and never coming back." These expressions are describing a reaction to the emotion, not the emotion. If you find yourself doing this, take a moment to examine what you have said. Beneath the action will be the true emotion.

Throughout this chapter, emphasis has been placed on focusing your attention inward. In order to become accustomed to feeling your emotions, you must accustom yourself to placing your awareness on what is going on inside you. Most of the time we are so busy paying attention to the outside world, we know very little about ourselves. It takes practice to notice what is going on inside. If you can learn to do this, while at the same time notice what is going on outside you, then you will begin to take charge of your life. You'll begin to react differently to the events in your life. You will begin to notice what you do that attracts particular experiences. You will know the emotion that causes it. You will learn to take responsibility for everything in your life. In taking responsibility, you will know how to change your life and make it the way you desire. You will know how to use your thoughts, and emotions, in compliance with your soul, to make permanent changes.

14

Working with Energy

All day long, we work with our energy fields. Most of the time, we don't even realize it. Just like a heart beating, our energy fields pulse. They expand and contract. Thoughts and emotions cause them to grow larger or smaller, change shapes and change colors. In this chapter I am going to explain some of the subconscious things we do that enhance, disturb, manipulate, and change our energy fields. The purpose of this explanation is to illustrate different approaches we can take to use our energy fields to our greatest advantage.

Going with the Flow: Using Our Energy Field to Its Greatest Advantage

Through my years of working with people, I found an optimum approach to living that creates a better flow of energy in the body. This approach also leads to the most incredible spiritual awakenings. Unfortunately, this approach is rarely used, yet it is the simplest thing to do. It is to say 'yes' to everything that happens.

Reacting to life by saying 'yes' puts you in total agreement with your soul, and the tools you were born with, your DNA. According to the System For Soul Memory, your soul is using the energy of your body to direct your life. It is directing you to think and feel in a certain way. It is also attracting specific events and people into your life so you can gain wisdom and know who you are. When you say 'yes' to the soul, you are telling the soul that you understand what the soul is doing. You acknowledge who is really in charge.

When you say 'yes', you are opening yourself up to learning something knew about yourself. You are allowing the energy that is coming from God to flow through you purely, without interruption. You are allowing an event to take place without trying to control it, stop it, reason it out, or excuse it.

Saying 'yes' to life sounds simple, but it is very difficult to accomplish. Saying 'yes' means you are willing to feel your emotions in the moment they occur. By saying 'yes', you are telling yourself that feeling your emotions is more important than reacting to a situation, or defending yourself. When you say yes, you are putting aside your ego for the sole purpose of spiritual awakening. Let me give you an example.

Let's say your lover has just told you that you hurt his or her feelings. Most people would respond by either denying it, or asking how or when they did such a thing. When you respond in this manner, you are *reacting* to the situation. You are thinking about what you did. You are plotting how to respond. You may be getting ready to defend yourself, reject the idea, or even walk away. If you are reacting to the situation, you are not saying 'yes.' You are doing everything but feeling the emotions the accusation has brought forth.

On the other hand, if you respond by saying, "Yes, if you say I hurt your feelings, then I must have," then you are allowing the emotional energy of the incident to be released. By releasing the energy, you are giving yourself the opportunity to explore the situation and observe your own feelings.

Saying yes validates the incident your soul just created to get you to feel an emotion. It brings forth the pain of hurting the one you love, and gives you the opportunity to feel the emotion behind it. Feeling the emotion creates immediate transcendence. In other words, feeling the emotion makes you instantly aware of why you did what you did. It allows you to know what you are thinking and what you are feeling. Having transcendence gives you the ability to gain the wisdom the soul desires. It allows you to validate the emotion of your lover, plus the emotion buried deep within your soul that is triggering the situation. Because of events in your childhood and other previous experiences, you wanted to hurt your lover's feelings. If you stop to feel the emotions you will know why you wanted to do this.

Once you feel the emotion and understand your subconscious motives, you will be able to say to your lover, "You are right. I did want to hurt you. I wanted to hurt you because I feel hurt. I feel hurt because...."

Saying 'yes' to your lover's emotions allows you to say 'yes' to your own emotions. When both parties are feeling their emotions, the most amazing thing happens. An ordinary event becomes a spiritual experience. Everyone's energy field expands and love permeates the situation.

When you can say yes to your actions and acknowledge the emotion and the deeper intent of the soul, you create the flow of energy to be as it should be, the way God intended it to be. When you do this, watch what happens, not just in your relationships, but in your life. Watch the healing that takes place. Watch how it filters through to everything in your life, even affecting strangers who come into contact with you. Saying 'yes' to life brings in so much loving energy, it puts you on the road to knowing ecstasy and rapture.

People are always asking me, "How can you stop in the middle of work to feel an emotion?" I do realize that sometimes it is difficult to give yourself fifteen minutes of alone time to process your emotions. If you can't do this, then there is something else you can do. Just notice the emotion that is surfacing. Be aware of what is going on inside you while you are reacting to what is going on outside you. Then later when you get home from work, take the time to process the emotion. The event will still be sharp in your mind and it will be easy to bring up the emotion again. Then process the emotion according to the steps of the System For Soul Memory. By being aware of the emotion when the event first happens makes it easy to feel it later.

Going Against the Flow: Manipulating Energy

Every time you stop the flow of emotion to react to a situation, you are manipulating energy. You are using your will power to bend, squelch, propel or distort the normal flow of energy through your chakras and around your body. This is done to gain control.

Everything is energy. And all energy is constantly moving. Energy moves because of the emotions that drive it. Therefore, when a situation occurs, there is a tremendous surge in the movement of energy. During this surge of energy, your brain operates on different levels as it evaluates the situation. It evaluates the information your five senses send you: the physical aspects of the situation, what you are seeing, hearing, touching, smelling or tasting. Plus the brain evaluates the information your energy field sends you: what you are feeling emotionally and intuitively. Most of the time, the information your energy field sends you is ignored and processed on a subconscious level. The only conscious inkling you will have, will be the feeling that you have lost control. You will feel this way because the energy, as it aggressively surges through you and at you, will throw you off balance. It will distort, and unsettle your energy field until you can make the necessary adjustments to rebalance yourself. If you rebalance yourself by evaluating the situation in terms of your emotions, you will be allowing for the optimum flow of energy. In other words, you will be rebalancing yourself directly through your energy field. If you rebalance yourself by reacting physically or mentally to the situation, then you will be stifling and manipulating the flow of energy. You will be rebalancing yourself through your five senses, and ignoring the disturbance of energy around you, which is sending you so much more information.

In terms of seeing this in the aura, the colors of the aura radiate with neon-bright light and the aura expands to more than twice its size when you respond by feeling your emotions. When you respond by manipulating energy, by thinking and reacting physically, the colors in the aura dim and the energy field shrinks.

Exercise:

To observe how you are affected by the energy around you, do this exercise. Before you walk into a room filled with people, stop for a moment to sense how you are feeling. Are you happy, sad, feel good about yourself, feel cranky, etc.? How do you feel physically? Once you know, walk into the room and notice immediately the next feeling assaulting you. Do not use your eyes for this experiment! Don't let what you see influence your feelings. Allow your chakras and your energy field to read the energy in the room for you. You may be amazed at how the energy in the room affects you. You may feel the emotions others are projecting towards you. Or you may feel drained as others rob energy from you. For example, if you were happy before walking into the room, then feel uncomfortable and sad just after you do, you are picking up the energy of the people in the room.

Also, inanimate objects, which are really animated objects of moving energy complete with consciousness—thoughts and feelings, absorb the energy of those around them, just like we do. To observe the difference in energy, notice how you feel when you walk into a toy store like FAO Schwarz where thousands of children have deposited their energy of happiness. Compare this to how you feel walking into a hospital, where thousands of sick people have deposited their energy of sadness, anger, and unprocessed emotions.

People learn to manipulate their energy in different ways. I will write about the few I have witnessed. I can always feel when people manipulate their energy. To me, the energy they put out always has a restrictive feel to it.

DNA is an important factor in what you do with your energy. You inherit the different ways you manipulate energy. These methods are then reinforced growing up. What your parents did with their energy taught you what to do with yours. If your parents were addictive and used physical substances to keep from feeling their emotions, then you will learn to do the same thing. If your parents tried to control their emotions by rationalizing everything, then you will do that too.

Manipulating energy leads to stress. If you take a moment to think about it, you can see why. Energy pulses and flows naturally through the chakras and around the body. When you begin to manipulate it by not wanting to think a certain thought, or by not wanting to feel a certain emotion, or by forcing your will to make something happen, then you are fighting against the natural flow of energy. Think of it as creating dams in a river and changing the flow of water. Wherever you create your dams, you create stress and tension in the flow of water. Wherever you manipulate the flow of energy in your body, you do the same thing. You create stress.

Where your parents held their stress in their body, is most likely the place where you will hold yours. I remember one day standing in the presence of a father who held all his stress in his Navel Chakra. I could feel it as a pressing feeling on my Navel Chakra. He was telling me that his daughter was suffering from Crohns disease, a disease of the intestines. His daughter learned to hold her stress in the same location, but took it one step further. I wasn't surprised. I learned that children are very sensitive to the energy fields around them, and will manipulate their energy fields to mimic those of their parents, or those closest to them.

If you want to know where you dam the flow of energy in your body, just find those areas in your body where you carry stress. For some people it's in their lower back, their Root Chakra, where, chances are, money problems are getting them down. For others, it's in the back of the neck, their Moon Center Chakra, where responsibilities are overpowering them. For some it's in the stomach, the Solar Plexus Chakra, where they are feeling powerless to something in their life. Find the area where you are carrying stress, and you will find the chakra where you are trying to manipulate the energy. To relieve the stress, you will need to take a moment to observe your body, then your life, to discover those issues and emotions you are trying to avoid or to control.

Manipulating Energy Through the Use of the Defense Drama

There are different ways energy is manipulated. One way energy is manipulated is through a **defense drama**.

A defense drama is a play that is created and acted out to avoid feeling an emotion. It is a specific routine of actions created by an individual that allows them to get caught up in the story of their life, so they don't have to feel the emotion underlying it.

The motivation for a defense drama will be generated by a strong emotion on a subconscious level. Many times, people will be aware of their actions, but not aware of the motivation causing their actions. The term 'defense' is used, because on a conscious level people feel the need to defend themselves against others. Yet on a subconscious level, what they are really doing is defending themselves against their own emotions.

The best way to explain a defense drama would be to give you an example of one. Allison is twenty-five years old. Her parents were divorced when she was sixteen. To this day, Allison has yet to feel the emotion of rejection the divorce created. Whenever the feeling of rejection surfaces, Allison uses her defense drama to protect herself. Her defense drama always involves pitting two other people against each other and goes like this.

Allison was supposed to meet her father for lunch, but he canceled at the last minute because of a business commitment. Allison, instead of feeling rejected, told her father that it was okay, that she understood. That night while talking to her mother, Allison told her what her father did. Then she told her mother that her father just bought his new wife a fur coat. Subconsciously, Allison knew this information would rile her mother, because her father's cheapness was one of the major contentions of their divorce. This created a heated exchange between her parents several weeks later. Allison's defense drama worked perfectly. Instead of feeling rejected, she managed to manipulate her mother into punishing her father for her.

Allison did all this without even realizing it. She does this in all areas of her life. If she feels one friend is getting too close to another, she will create a little drama to pit one against the other. At work, if one colleague is being favored over her, she will use her boss to do the same thing. All this is done subconsciously. Allison learned to manipulate energy in this manner from her mother while she was growing up.

Another type of defense drama is a phobia or a panic attack. This type of drama is based on an incident of extreme terror that occurred in the first eight years of life. The energy of the terror continues to get buried, distorted and manipulated until later it develops into the drama of a phobia or a panic attack. Take for example the case of Suzanne. When she was five her parents took her to an amusement park where they took her for a ride on the giant roller coaster. As an adult Suzanne suffered from fear of heights. She wasn't even able to drive over a bridge without sweating and feeling the terror. When Suzanne was finally able to walk through the terror, she saw the seed pattern where the emotion first originated. It was on the roller coaster ride when she was five. In talking to people, I discovered amusement parks to be a common seed pattern for panic attacks and phobias in adults.

When you are being obsessive or compulsive you are also creating a defense drama to act out an emotion instead of feel it. For some people who were taught to fear their emotions, it is easier to wash their hands 30 times a day than to feel the emotion underlying it.

Manipulating Energy by Projecting Your Energy onto Others

Another way energy is manipulated is by projecting your unwanted energy onto someone else. In other words, making them feel the emotion you don't want to feel yourself. Take the case of Burt. Growing up, Burt never felt as smart as his brother or his sister. Competition was keen on who made better grades in school. Burt's father was always quick to praise the one who did better. Burt was rarely praised. Burt earned a Master's degree in English, but that wasn't enough. Burt continued his studies until he received a Master's degree in Social Work, too. Burt became a teacher. When Burt met Elizabeth, a new teacher in the school, he fell head over heels in love. After they dated for a while, Elizabeth broke up with him. Her reason: he criticized her too much. "You make me feel like I'm not good enough, that I'm stupid," she told him. I am a well-educated woman, yet when I'm around you, I feel stupid."

When someone projects their unwanted emotions towards you, chances are they are mirroring a similar buried emotion within you. After all, like energy attracts like energy. You will know if the emotion they are projecting towards you is your issue too, by what you feel later. If what they said or did continues to linger in your thoughts well after the incident took place, then you share the issue.

Manipulating Energy: Creating Physical Problems in the Body

Sometimes to keep from feeling an emotion, people will manipulate their energy field in such a way that they create a physical problem in the body. I discovered this to be true in a wide range of circumstances, from cases of extreme abuse, to a simple matter of not wanting to listen to a parent. Some people, through determination and will power, will go to extreme measures in using the energies of their bodies to protect themselves.

For example, while I had my bookstore, a psychologist came in and ordered a book about multiple personalities. We spoke briefly about the subject, since this was her specialty. Three weeks later, an article appeared in the local newspaper that detailed the increased number of cases of multiple personalities in my area. The article went on to describe the problem in full including the symptoms of the disorder. Later that day, while I was working, a young woman and her friends, walked into my store to ask me a question about 'out of body' experiences. She explained to me how she would wake up in the morning and wouldn't remember anything until later in the afternoon. She would go out with her friends and not remember being with them. They piped in and explained different scenarios. She asked me if this was happening because she was having 'out of body experiences.' As soon as I saw this girl, I knew intuitively that she had been badly abused as a child. I also knew that it was no coincidence that I had met the psychologist or brought to the store that article I had read in the morning paper about multiple personalities. So when I asked her what other names she called herself, and she and her friends told me, I also knew that I was going to feel what she did with the energy waves of her brain to keep herself from feeling her emotions. Because of my psychic ability I felt how she altered her brain waves to change personalities when an emotion surfaced. It felt like a switch being turned on, rerouting the information, like the switch on a railroad track that sends the train heading into another direction. I gave the young woman the newspaper article and the business card for the psychologist. When I saw her again a month later, she told me that she felt much better now that she understood her problem. Unfortunately, she saw the psychologist only once, because she couldn't afford the therapy.

I was also in the presence of someone having a nervous breakdown. This man came into my store thinking that a psychic could help him. I discovered that many times, people who prefer to stay in denial about their emotions would rather see a psychic than a therapist. This man was having panic attacks and unwanted thoughts. He wanted to know if a spirit possessed him. Intuitively I was feeling that he was having a nervous breakdown. I could feel the energy of his brain going on overload. I sensed his unwanted thoughts were a deeply buried memory of a long ago trauma filled with terror and sexual abuse, which he later confirmed. While his brain was working hard to uncover the memory, he was trying to suppress the overpowering flow of emotion and terror that surfaced with it. He was trying to do everything with his brain, which wasn't in a normal functioning mode as it worked to release the buried memory. I could feel his terror, plus I could feel the absence of stability in not having the brain working in a normal functioning mode. It felt like the man was disintegrating, flying apart. I told him he needed to see a doctor. He came back a few months later and described his breakdown and his stay in a mental health facility. He told me the doctor gave him drugs to stop the overpowering flow of emotion.

In each of these cases, emotions were constantly suppressed and not dealt with. These people tried controlling their energy, their thoughts and emotions, with their brain. They used determination and will power to do this. In both cases the brain finally broke down and rebelled, causing their mental disorders.

Yet I found when other people used the System For Soul Memory to deal with long buried childhood traumas, and concentrated on their emotions in the chakras instead of what is going on in their brain, they were able to get through the traumatic memories without drugs. When reliving a trauma such as this from the past, you will remember it as though you are a child again. You won't have the added knowledge and wisdom of your adulthood to get you through it. You will experience it from the distorted viewpoint of a child who can't make sense out of what is happening. That is why there is so much terror. The pictures will be hazy and not always accurate, but the emotions will be. As the trauma comes to light, your whole body will be affected. You may suffer flu-like symptoms, feel nauseous and jittery, and even throw up. I saw people affected in this manner. I experienced it myself.

Warning! I wish to state emphatically if you are experiencing something similar, and you need assistance, please seek the aid of a qualified professional. Some people are able to do this on their own. Others need assistance. No matter what you do, whether you use drugs or not, you still have to walk through your emotions and the feelings of terror in order to heal.

A learning disability is another example where the flow of energy gets distorted and creates a physical condition in the body. I found this generally to exist in a person who uses their brain to block out something in their life that makes them feel powerless. Instead of feeling the emotion, they distort the brain chemistry to create a block so they won't have to deal with it. I witnessed this during counseling sessions. For example, the spiritual counseling session with Rachel was going fine until I mentioned a long ago trauma. This triggered a buried emotion to surface. Not wanting to deal with the emotion, Rachel's learning disability went into action. Rachel's learning disability had to do with not being able to process what she hears. As soon as I felt her energy begin to restrict me, I knew she was manipulating her energy field and would no longer hear what I was going to say. So I confronted her with this. She had no idea she was creating the learning disability. Yet, once she became aware of what she was doing, she was able to change the pattern.

Another example of manipulating the body's energy is to make yourself sick. When Jane was five and started school, her mother started working full time. Jane felt the loss of love dramatically. During her first month of school, Jane came down with a bad case of the flu. Her mother was forced to stay home and care for her. Jane loved that her mother was home again and giving her so much attention. On a subconscious level, Jane associated being sick as a way to receive attention. Jane continued to use this pattern growing up. When she married and felt ignored because her husband was too busy working, she got sick. Consciously, she had no idea she was creating her illnesses because of an association she made as a child, or that she was creating it to mask the emotion of feeling lonely. When her husband became immune to her constant little illnesses, Jane became even sicker to attract his attention. It wasn't until the emotion became so deeply buried and manifested as cancer that Jane was finally forced to confront her actions.

Manipulating Energy: Using a Physical Substance or a Physical Sensation to Feel an Emotion

The most common manipulation of energy is addiction. I find that people who are addicted have learned to feel their emotions through a physical substance or sensation. Being addicted to alcohol, drugs, smoking, working, sex, food, or gambling, is a genetic and a learned trait. People who are addicted don't know how to feel their emotions emotionally. In fact, these people are so far removed from their emotions, that in working with those who are in recovery and in teaching them the System For Soul Memory, I discovered that it generally takes them a year to feel an emotion the way it was meant to be felt. These people are very sensitive, and intuitive. Growing up in a chaotic home teaches them to use all their resources. Many of them are quick to tell me that they feel too much, that is why they seek solace in their addiction. Yet when I am talking to them and an emotion surfaces, they don't know what to do with it. They describe the emotion in physical terms. For example instead of knowing they are feeling the emotion of abandonment, they describe it as a heavy pressing feeling on their chest. Confusing emotions with the physical is why they are able to bury their emotions in their addiction.

Children who grow up with someone in the family, who is addicted, only know an addictive kind of love. This kind of love has an obsessive quality to it and usually works from extremes. It is unreliable, the love being there one minute, then gone the next. And it is unpredictable going from super-loving and smothering one moment, to being filled with rage and violence the next. It can also be quite controlling or the opposite, quite unstable or chaotic. So the first time in the first eight years a child begins to feel the loss of love by an addictive parent, will determine how the child's addiction will surface later in his life. In the development of the chakras, there is a pattern to the addiction. What type of addiction a child suffers later in life will depend at what age he or she first suffered through the trauma of being loved like this.

If a child senses this lack of love in the first two years during the development of the Root Chakra and the Navel Chakra, the child's addiction will reflect in one of four ways: either through gambling, sex, eating, or being a workaholic.

If a child feels lack of love between the ages of four and five, during the development of the Heart Chakra and the Throat Chakra, then his addiction will be through alcoholism or smoking.

The Solar Plexus Chakra is like a bridge. If the child feels lack of love during the age of three when this chakra develops, then his addiction will be at least one addiction from both groups of chakras just below and above. In other words, he will suffer with the addiction of gambling, sex, overworking, or eating; and he will suffer with the addiction of drinking or smoking. (See Diagram 3)

If a child feels lack of love between the ages of seven and eight during the development of the Third Eye Chakra and the Crown Chakra, then his addiction will manifest through using a controlled substance like marijuana, crack, cocaine, heroine, and prescription drugs.

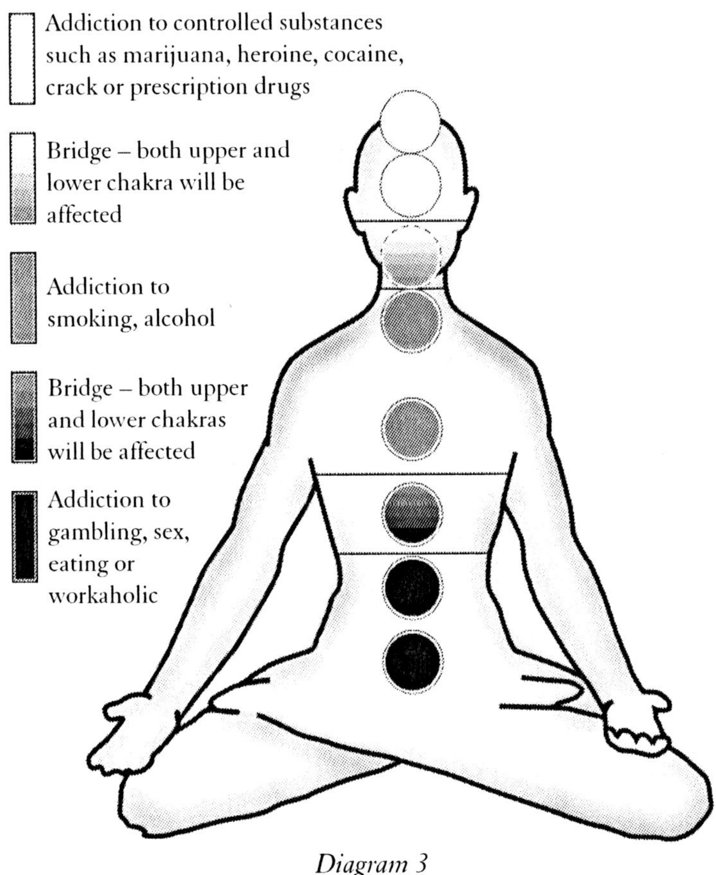

Diagram 3

The Moon Center Chakra is another bridge. If the child feels lack of love during the age of six when this chakra develops, then his addiction will be at least one addiction from both groups of chakras just below and above. He will do both: smoke or drink, and take drugs.

Unfortunately, I found the love in the homes of addicted people to be so chaotic that most addicted people suffer from more than one addiction. It is not unusual for them to give up one addiction only to begin suffering with another. Yet at the center is the emotion of feeling unloved. As I stated previously, addicted people don't know how to feel unloved. They only know how to live it. They prove daily that they are unlovable. They do this by either harming themselves with their addictions, or by finding others to do it for them. Their parents taught them that love hurts and they continue the defense drama they were taught by hurting themselves through their addiction.

Working with Energy: Energy Stimulators

While working with people and learning about energy and emotions, I discovered three emotions that are more potent in moving energy than other emotions. I call these emotions **energy stimulators**. They are anger, desire and will.

I also call these emotions **surface emotions** because they are the emotions that lay on the surface of almost every other emotion. They are the emotions that push the other emotions to the forefront, and they are the emotions you experience first.

When you want to make changes in your life these are the three emotions you call forth to help make those changes. These emotions reside in different chakras and they all create change, but with different consequences.

Anger

When something doesn't work right is when you notice you want it changed. Anger is the emotion most widely used to make changes. Anger is found in the Solar Plexus Chakra. This is the chakra where energy is created. Energy coming from this chakra is one of the most explosive of all the emotions. In Chapter 13, I stated that it is very hard to sit still and feel anger. Anger wants you to move.

When anger appears, it generally means you feel you've been hurt. You were either victim or passive to something in your life. Energy came from an outside source and attacked you. The usual response is to lash back.

Most people call anger destructive. Anger as we know it today is being misused. It is not being felt, but is being acted upon instead. Most people act out their anger rather than feel it. Acting out anger means to be physical with it. To slam doors, break things, yell, or the worst scenario, hurt others with it. Most of the violence in our world comes from anger being acted out. Yet when anger is used positively, it is a good energy source for making changes in your life.

Because anger is such a powerful energy, when it is stifled, it creates a distortion in the energy field in your body. When I see it in an aura, it shows itself as being a muddied red. People with cancer have auras that are a muddied red. Therefore, I concluded that too much stifled anger is the energy stimulator that leads to cancer.

Will

Will is another emotion used to make changes. Will sits in the Third Eye Chakra, the chakra that holds your belief systems. Will is the emotion used when you want to stifle a surfacing emotion. Will is also the emotion used when you want to implement an idea or create something new. The emotional energy of will puts your thoughts into action.

Will can also help you overcome obstacles and perform miracles. Will is the energy stimulator that creates the expression "mind over matter."

Yet using will can have its drawbacks, especially if it is used too often to avoid dealing with an emotion. Will gives you the false sense that you have control over your life, because by exerting your will, you can do what you want. Yet as you have learned, the soul is really in charge. No matter how much will you use to make your life the way you *think* you want it, the soul will show you how you really want it *emotionally*.

When anger is used, you feel you have been hurt. When will is used, you hurt others. You are forcing your energy onto others to get what you want. You are manipulating your energy and theirs.

Using too much will eventually distorts the energy of the brain. People, who go overboard in using their will to try and control their world and their emotions, are people who end up with brain problems such as headaches, migraines, tumors and strokes.

Desire

Desire is the least used energy stimulator. Desire resides in the Heart Chakra and comes from a place of love. There are no consequences when desire is used. Desire comes from the soul. God intended that energy be manipulated in this manner to get what you want.

The more you love yourself, the easier it is to have what you want through the desire of it. What do I mean by loving yourself? By feeling all your emotions. In feeling your emotions you are agreeing with God and saying I love how I am. This creates an incredible flow of energy around the body. This flow of energy attracts everything. Think of it as a giant magnet. When you love yourself, you draw everything to you. Everything gets attracted to love.

The soul remembers everything you have ever desired, and brings it to you. The soul also remembers all the stigmas, hurts, and past attachments you have connected to your desire. Until you can clear all the past hurts that block you from having what you want, you won't realize your desire. If you are slow to process your emotions, expect it to take years for your desire to manifest.

Working with Energy: Things You Can Do to Increase the Energy of Your Body

Through working with people and seeing auras, I discovered certain activities you can do that will increase the size of your aura and make it glow with stronger light. When your aura is stronger and brighter, you feel better, your life flows more easily, and it's easier to manifest what you want.

I'm sure I have omitted other activities that can increase the level of energy in your aura. The purpose of this list is to make you aware of what you do in your daily life and how it affects your energy field. You will know in your own life what electrifies your energy field. It will make you feel good, and increase your level of wellness.

1. Feel your emotions
2. Pray
3. Meditate
4. Breathe deeply
5. Be creative
6. Sing—chant
7. Do the things that make you happy
8. Laugh
9. Exercise
10. Spend time with nature or animals

Working with Energy: Things You Do That Stifle the Flow of Energy in Your Body

Below is a list of things you do that crimps the flow of energy in the body. In watching people's auras while they did these things, I noticed their auras shrink and the colors become muddied, muted and dimmed. People generally felt drained afterwards. Also the more you do the following things, the more depressed you will feel. The continued stifling of energy always leads to accidents, and illness. Eventually when there is no more energy feeding the body, death occurs.

1. Don't feel your emotions
2. Act out your feelings
3. Rationalize

4. Feel Guilty
5. Judge yourself: lie, cheat, steal, be morally wrong, unethical, feel unworthy, undeserving, etc.
6. Judge others
7. Do things when you don't want to do them
8. Be responsible when you don't want to be

Exercise:

Take a moment to observe your life. Look at the list of things that increase the flow of energy. How many of these things do you do each day? Now look at the list of things that decrease your energy. How many of these things do you do each day? In my experience most people do more that decreases their energy, than increases their energy.

15

How to Use Your Energy System to Get What You Want

Once you understand how your energy system works, you can use it to help you get the things in life you want. In this chapter, I am going to explain once again the fundamental principles of energy based on the System For Soul Memory, and show you how you can use these principles to manifest what you want. Let's reiterate what we have learned so far about energy.

The Principles of Energy According to the System for Soul Memory

1. For every action there is an equal reaction. Therefore, every time you create the energy of I want, you create the energy of I don't want.
2. Like energy attracts like energy. According to your soul, everything you want is in your life at this exact moment. If you desire something and it is not in your life, then to your soul, you don't want it; therefore, you haven't attracted it.

3. Each chakra carries with it a specific theme and function. Knowing how to understand the energy of each chakra will explain why you are creating the life you attract.
4. During the first eight years of your life, during the development of each chakra and the development of your seed patterns, your belief system is established. This belief system determines how you manifest what you want.
5. You must use the principle of transcendence in order to move energy and manifest what you want. The principle of transcendence relies on using the combination of the physical, the emotional and the mental in order to gain wisdom and realize a result on the subatomic level of the soul. In terms of using transcendence to manifest what you want, you must know *physically* what you want. Secondly, you must use *emotion* to trigger the energy and get the manifestation process moving. And third, you must have *mental* awareness of the manifestation process.

We know that for every action there is an equal reaction. As soon as the energy of good is created, so too is the energy of bad. This also applies to what you want. As soon as you create the energy of 'I want,' you also create the energy of 'I don't want.' In terms of the soul, polarity is basic. It is the way energy is compared, measured, and evaluated.

In terms of manifesting, you won't know what you want unless you know what you don't want. What this means is that every time you say you want something, you will also manifest what you don't want so that your soul can compare and *know* the difference. The soul does this to gain the wisdom.

Generally, we are already living with the 'I don't want' attitude. In other words, if what you desire is not in your life at the present time, then you are living with the 'I don't want' attitude. What is buried in your subconscious is manifesting this condition. In order to change this pattern of energy you must first validate it.

You must discover why you don't want it, then you must feel the emotion that is triggering it.

You already know why you want something. To discover why you don't want it will be more difficult. But there are different methods you can use that will help you discover the reason.

First look at your beliefs. What do you believe about the item that you want? What are your overall beliefs about having things? Generally these are the beliefs your parents drilled into you growing up.

Some of the common beliefs I heard over the years are:

1. You don't get things for free.
2. You have to work for what you want.
3. Money doesn't grow on trees.
4. Waste not, want not.
5. The things in life that are worthwhile don't come easily.
6. You get what you pay for.

These are just a few of the standard beliefs we hear growing up which we take to heart. They become the beliefs by which we live. Look at your life and see which beliefs you manifest. Then you will see why you create struggle. Every belief I mentioned above creates struggle. We make those beliefs come true.

For example, when Keith was five, he wanted a bike for Christmas. He told his parents what he wanted. They said nothing, so Keith assumed he was going to get what he desired. When Christmas morning came and Keith ran to the Christmas tree, instead of finding a bike, he found some new sneakers, a sweater and a new jacket. Disappointed, Keith confronted his parents. "Why didn't you buy me a bike? I wanted a bike. Not these stupid clothes." Keith's parents were having money troubles that year and couldn't afford to spend money on the nonessentials. Feeling humiliated at their failure, and at Keith's disappointment, they lashed out at him, "Money doesn't grow on trees! Be thankful for what you got." Keith always remembered the incident as one of humiliation and guilt. His subconscious belief was 'Because money doesn't grow on trees, it's humiliating to ask for something. As an adult, Keith manifested this belief in his job. Wherever he worked, whenever he would ask his boss for a raise, his boss would respond negatively by humiliating him and telling him how times were hard for the company, and that he should be thankful for what he had.

To look at this from a different perspective, take the case of Joey. When Joey was five, his church was holding a raffle. The grand prize was a new bike. Joey's mother bought him a ticket and told him. "Joey, you can win. If you want something badly enough, you can have it." Joey won the bike. As an adult, people always thought Joey was lucky. His life seemed easy. But Joey always told people, "I'm not lucky. You just have to want something bad enough and you can have it."

Your belief patterns are comprised of what you think and feel. These belief patterns originated in the first eight years of your life. In order to change these patterns, you must delve into your subconscious and discover why you think and feel the way you do. You must go back to the first eight years of your life and remember what was said, what you did, what was done to you, and what you felt, in order to understand why you have the beliefs you do. There will always be a logical reason.

Sometimes it is very difficult to discover the subconscious reason why you can't manifest what you want. Either the memory is too deeply buried, or the belief is too obvious you have trouble seeing it. If this happens, there is a 'game' you can play that will trick you into discovering the true reason for your lack. This game relaxes the defensive wall your conscious mind erects and allows the subconscious to come through and give you the reason.

Exercise:

Say aloud, "I don't want ____ (the thing you crave most) ____ because...." Begin to list the reasons why you don't want it. Immediately, your conscious mind will fight you. It will tell you that you are being ridiculous; that what you are saying is false, because you do want that object. So in the beginning you are going to play a game and 'lie' to yourself. You are going to make up reasons. For the exercise to work, you should think up reasons that are ridiculous and fun. The more ridiculous you try to make the answers, the more it frees your conscious mind to let go.

Your left brain rules your conscious mind. This is the thinking and processing side of your brain. Your right brain is where you are creative and intuitive. It is where your inspiration comes from, and it is your connection to your soul. When you begin making up reasons, you are accessing the right side of your brain and the ability to know your subconscious. The most amazing thing happens while you are playing this game. The real reason will suddenly slip out. You will know it because it will come through as a burst of emotion or an expansion of sudden insight. Like having an epiphany. Then you will know why you don't have what you crave most in your life.

For example, Melissa wants a new car. Her car is ten years old and she can't afford to buy a new one. When I tell Melissa she doesn't really want a new car since she doesn't have the means to get one, she immediately flies into a burst of denial. So I tell her that if she really did want a new car, it would be in her life now. Many people have trouble understanding this philosophy. Yet this philosophy is another example of how energy works. Like energy attracts like energy. If Melissa radiated the energy of desiring a new car, she would have attracted the car into her life. Since she doesn't have a new car, she is not radiating that energy. Obviously, on the level of the soul, Melissa doesn't want a new car. To find out why, I got Melissa to play the game. Melissa's reasons went as follows:

I don't want a new car because that means I would have to worry about where I park it.

I don't want a new car because the first time I got a ding or a dent I would really be upset.

I don't want a new car because my old car still drives fine and I would feel guilty getting rid of something that was still good.

At this point I stopped Melissa and asked her where that belief came from. She told me from her father who worked very hard his whole life to provide for them. I asked her if that brought up an emotion, which it did, in her Moon Center Chakra. I asked her to hone in on it. This helped her to remember what happened at six years old. She remembered throwing out a perfectly good knapsack she no longer wanted. Her father saw her do this and got very upset with her. He made her feel guilty and ashamed because he said she was spoiled and didn't deserve to have such nice things. Melissa cried and felt the buried emotions. She felt her father was too hard on her. After all, she was only six and didn't understand. In feeling the old buried emotions, she realized why she didn't want the new car. She was still carrying around the old feelings of guilt that she was spoiled and didn't deserve to have it.

Melissa called me back three weeks later to tell me she got a new car. Her parents decided to retire and move to Florida. They were giving her their year-old, four-wheel drive because they didn't think they would need it anymore.

Sometimes you think you want something when on later reflection you realize you really don't. It is only your soul trying to get you to clear an old buried emotion. For example, Roger wants a date with Ellen. She has turned him down repeatedly. In speaking to Roger, he didn't believe me when I told him that he was the one telling Ellen to turn him down. So I got Roger to play the game with me. Here were his reasons for not wanting a date with Ellen:

I don't want to go out with Ellen because it means I would have to wash and wax my car.

I don't want to go out with Ellen because it means I would have to buy a new suit.

I don't want to go out with Ellen because she would want to go to the movies and then I would have to sit through two hours of a boring, silly movie.

I don't want to go out with Ellen because I would have to spend money.

I don't want to go out with Ellen because she reminds me of Jill who lived next door to me when I was little.

As soon as Roger said this, I stopped him. He was shocked at what he said. I then asked him to tell me about Jill. Did he have any negative thoughts about her? Roger explained that Jill's father was alcoholic. Roger always heard yelling and screaming coming from their house. He felt bad for Jill but there was nothing he could do. He remembered treating her poorly, teasing her and being mean, no different than how the rest of the kids in the neighborhood treated her. Later as an adult, he always regretted treating her so poorly because he knew she had a hard life. Roger realized Ellen had the same kind of energy. He must have been picking up subconsciously that Ellen came from the same kind of background as Jill. Roger later called me after he discovered this was true. He told me he no longer desired to go out with her. He realized that he had attracted Ellen into his life to heal his old buried guilt about Jill.

Whatever you desire you will manifest, even if it is not manifested right away. Every thought, every feeling and every desire you have gets written in your soul. The soul remembers everything and attracts it into your life for you.

When your energy field is fully activated and free of emotional blocks you will be able to manifest anything you want instantly. That is the sign of an enlightened master, or someone with a fully realized brain, like Jesus or Sai Baba. Emotional blocks prevent you from having what you want. How quickly you manifest will tell you how blocked your energy field is. As soon as you desire something, your soul will show you what those emotional blocks are. If it takes you a year to get it, then that is how long it took you to feel all the buried emotions creating the block. If on the other hand you manifest right away, then your energy pattern was relatively clear. To get what you want, you must be willing to deal with the blocks when the soul reveals them to you.

In my meditations, I was shown how energy attracts. It is love that is doing the attracting. Everything in the universe wants to be loved. People who love profoundly draw to them everything in the universe. They attract everything they desire. And what do I mean by people who love themselves? These are people who are free of self-judgment, who allow themselves to feel every emotion God gave them as a learning experience. Because they have felt their own pain they are not afraid to feel the pain of others. Feeling other people's pain is the greatest way they demonstrate their love. They never judge what others do; instead they feel compassion for their plight and what they have gone through. That is why they attract everyone and everything to them. Jesus was the perfect example of this. People ran to him wanting to be touched by his love. Everything in the universe stood ready waiting to fulfil his slightest command. When he took on the sins of others and healed them, what he was really doing was feeling their guilt and shame and the emotions they were too afraid to feel.

All energy wants to be validated. It wants to be recognized and loved. When you have an emotion that you deny or won't validate, the soul will bring it to your attention. It will create problems for you until you finally stop and validate it. That is why it is good to stop for a minute and validate your life and what you have created in it. Validate all the negativity you attract. Until you do you will not be able to change it.

Transcendence in the Manifestation Process

There are two ways you manifest things in your life. There is the human approach in which you think of the thing you want then go out and physically get it yourself.

Or there is the energy approach where you simply desire it and without any physical exertion, it comes to you. As I mentioned before, this approach uses energy to manifest. It requires the principles of transcendence. As I stated previously, Eastern religions believe that when you are in a state of transcendence, you are accessing your spirit, God. Only in this state can you move energy and change things.

Therefore, there are three things you must do to make your manifestation process work.

1. You must have a good physical picture or idea of what it is you wish to manifest.
2. You must use emotion to move the energy to make it happen. Remember that emotion triggers the movement of energy. Desire, which is born from love, is the most powerful emotion to use in the manifestation process. Yet any emotion will work.
3. You must have mental awareness of the process. In other words, you must validate every step of the journey. Not only must you be aware of what you want, you must also be aware of why you don't want it. You must be aware of every thought, feeling, and belief system that prohibits you from attaining your desire.

I find it interesting, that when asked, most people don't know what it is they want. They usually know what they don't want. Therefore, before using your energy system to get what you want, I recommend spending time and really thinking about what it is you want. Make a list. See if you can fill the list with ten items. Also make a list of the things in your life you wish to change. This will force you to make clear your desires and enable you to know where to direct your energies.

To start the manifestation process you must first be specific in what it is you want. You must be able to picture it clearly in your mind. You can't just say you want money. Money is a tool to buy things. It is a trigger just as emotion is. It gets things moving on a physical level just as emotion gets things moving on an energy level. You will never have what you want if you ask for money. Instead, you must know the object that you desire.

Once you picture what it is you want, then you must feel yourself wanting it. Feel yourself desiring it. Or if you picture yourself falling in love, imagine yourself with someone and feel yourself being in love and being loved in return. Or if you want a new job, picture yourself working at something you love doing and feel yourself being happy doing it. This starts the manifestation process. Once you use emotion you are speaking to the soul in the language that it knows. You are telling the soul, this is what I want.

Once you tell the soul this is what I want, the soul then shows you why you don't want it. It starts reminding you of painful memories and old hurts. It creates situations to reflect these emotions back to you. It will show you how your beliefs interfere with what you want. When you begin the manifestation process, be prepared. You must stay mentally aware of what you are creating and why. You must be sure to feel all the emotions that surface. You must be open to changing any attitudes that will prohibit your desire from manifesting.

Using the Chakras to Help You Manifest

Some books will recommend meditating on the chakras to help you get what you want. For people who are first learning to feel their emotions fully, I do not recommend doing this. Meditating on the chakras may unleash a flurry of painful memories you are not ready to handle. It could aggravate sudden illness or create life-changing situations. I have seen this happen many times, especially with people who use the chakras for healing energy work. If you do energy work and your life is in chaos, you are not using energy correctly.

You do not need to meditate on the chakras. All you have to do is tell the soul what you desire, and the soul will gladly show you what lies buried in your chakras. The soul knows what you can handle and what you can't. Therefore, you must have faith and patience in allowing the soul to manifest what you want at the rate it knows you can handle. For some people who choose denial and are slow to feel their emotions, getting what they want can take years.

Yet you can use what you know about your chakras to understand yourself better and why you don't manifest what it is you want. As I have written previously, each chakra vibrates to its own theme and performs certain functions. You can use this knowledge to discover your seed patterns, and your core beliefs. This will help you learn why you are not manifesting what it is you want. Here is a refined overview of what the chakras do.

The Root Chakra deals with survival and how your needs are met. This chakra helps create your physical world. Therefore, literally everything you own in your life will be a function of this chakra. This chakra will be critical if you wish to manifest something physical into your life like a home, a job, or anything money can buy. As stated in Chapter 5, what happened to you in the first year of life will determine how much you have.

The Navel Chakra helps you to make decisions. Unless you have a decision to make, you will not want to use this chakra for manifesting. The energy of this chakra is also passive and receptive, and not conducive for manifesting. It is generally a chakra where you feel like a victim, where you lay blame. If you are codependent and live to fulfill others needs, or if you do too much for others at your own expense, then you are spending too much time in this chakra. When you put out too much energy for others and you ignore yourself in the process, you distort your energy field. You tell the soul that others are more important than you are. Therefore, every time you tell the soul you want something, the soul then shows you how others should get it first. If you find you are doing this, then I always recommend that you begin acting more selfishly. People with this tendency will find this hard to do. Their energy field is so out of balance that what they think is selfish is really the normal mode of generosity for most people.

The Solar Plexus Chakra is the seat of your power. This is where energy is created. The more energy you create, the more you enhance your ability to manifest. Remember the different ways you build energy. First, the greatest way you build energy is through the soul, through feeling all your emotions, through feeling love. The second way is from prana, the subatomic energy found in the air we breathe. Many Eastern traditions such as yoga have excellent breathing techniques geared towards raising the energy of the body.

The third way is from the outside world: from other people, animals and nature. If your energy is lacking something, the soul will attract whatever it is you need. This not only applies to people, but to things in nature. You will crave certain foods, be attracted to certain gems and stones. You will want to take a walk through the woods, or by a beach. You will also attract certain types of animals. Maybe you will suddenly find mice in your home, or birds nesting closer to your house.

Insects are also incredible healers. Whatever insects you attract into your life are there to help you. Cockroaches are telling you that you are too overwhelmed by what is going on in your life; spiders, that you are feeling trapped in some way; mosquitoes, that you have an issue with getting something easily or for nothing. These are only a few. If you want to know why you have attracted a specific insect or animal, you only need to validate to your soul that you are aware of what you have attracted. Your soul will then inform you why it is in your life and tell you what it is that you are lacking. This knowing may not occur immediately and not in the way you may expect. Therefore, I always recommend that once you ask your soul a question, just let it go and not worry about it anymore. The answer will come to you when you least expect it. After all, your soul wants you to be happy and whole.

Become more aware of your energy field. Realize what things make you vibrate with more love and power and which things deplete you. Remember, by energy I do not mean how much physical pep you have. I am talking about your aura and the energy field that surrounds you.

Exercise:

A good way to measure your energy field is to put your hands together in front of you, palms flat, as though in a praying mode. Slowly draw your hands away from each other until they are as far apart as they can go. Keeping your attention focused on the palms of your hands, slowly begin to bring your hands back together. You will notice a point where you feel more resistance. This is where the energy field around each hand begins. As you learn to create more energy, you should notice how the space between your hands grows wider.

The Heart Chakra is where the energy of desire is created. Desire is based on love and is the most powerful tool you have to manifest. As I stated before, whatever you desire, and by desire I mean actually feeling it in your heart what it is you want, you will attract. The soul guarantees you this. Just be prepared for the manner in which the soul presents it to you. If you have definite expectations, the manifestation process will take longer. Each expectation will be no different than an interfering belief. The soul will have to remove them in order for your desire to be granted.

The Throat Chakra and the Moon Center Chakra deal with awareness of the self. These chakras help you establish your sense of self-esteem and feelings of self worth. Unless you feel good enough to have something, you will have trouble either having it or holding on to it. The soul will clearly demonstrate this to you. You may be given something only to lose it or have it taken away. If you notice this is happening to you, look back to the ages of five and six and see if something happened in your childhood that precipitated this.

The Throat Chakra gives you the ability to communicate on all levels. If you want to sing better, or have the ability to communicate better, then concentrate on this chakra. Find out where you have your blocks that prevent you from having success.

The Moon Center Chakra is the home of self-judgment and guilt, the biggest depressors of energy you can create. Therefore, when you decide you want something, check to see if you feel guilty or judgmental about having it. The more you judge or feel guilty, the more you stop the flow of energy and prevent yourself from having things.

This chakra is also the home of responsibility. If you are too responsible, in other words, if you hate what you are doing but do it because of a sense of responsibility, then you will have a hard time manifesting things. The soul wants you to be happy. Before you were born, God gave you a blueprint of the lessons you will learn, of the things you will want to do and have a talent doing. This will be evident in your DNA, and will show up as being your natural inclinations. This is God showing you what you should be doing. If you are not following this blueprint and not doing what you love, then you will create lack in your life. You will make your life more difficult.

Most people don't follow their natural inclinations. Family influence, events, or society turn them away from being their true selves. Each influence that turns them away is one of their learning lessons. Each one will have to be dealt with before they will know how to manifest easily.

The Third Eye Chakra is where your beliefs sit. Just look at your life at this moment, and you will see what you believe. If you find that your ideas are not easily accepted, then use this chakra to discover why. Also, this chakra is the home of your will, how determined you are.

The Crown Chakra is your God chakra. In other words, it is the chakra where you accept that you are God living the life of Jane or Bill, etc. By validating and accepting this blueprint God wants for you, you are creating the easiest, happiest and most peaceful life you can have. You clear all the blocks in your energy field so that you have direct communication with God.

When I think of this chakra, I think of the Yin/Yang symbol. (See Diagram 4) The white of the Crown Chakra, you-as-God-made-you chakra, joins forces with the black of the Root Chakra, you-as-human chakra, in a harmonious merging that enables you to manifest anything you want. Without the full acceptance of how God made you in your human existence you won't know ease. Without the full acceptance of how you are as human in your spiritual practices, you won't know God.

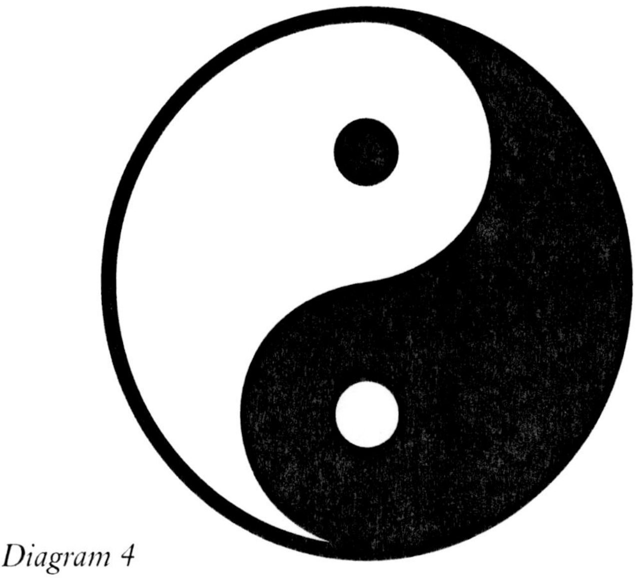

Diagram 4

Beliefs Concerning Money

Most people believe that money is the tool that gets them what they want. Therefore, I think it is important when talking about manifesting that you hone in on your beliefs about money. Take a moment to answer the following questions so that you can get clear on what your beliefs are.

1. **Where does money come from?** Your job, your boss, from God, your parents, your spouse, the Universe or from you? Look at what you create in your life and you will see what you really believe. In other words, if you believe that money only comes from your job, then you will create a life where the only money you get will be the money you work for. If you believe this, then forget about winning the lottery or getting things for free!

   For example: Naomi is twenty-eight, single and still living at home with her parents who are devout Jews. When I saw Naomi, she wanted to know if I saw a good paying job in her future. Naomi had been out of work for six months, and was having trouble finding a job that would pay her enough so that she could move into her own apartment. When I didn't see one, I asked Naomi where she thought money came from. She was quick to reply, "From God." Yet when I asked her further questions and got her to validate the reality of her life, she realized that on a subconscious level, she believed money came from her father. This caused several strong emotional issues to surface. By the time we finished speaking, Naomi saw how she was living her belief. The only money she was getting at the moment was coming from her father. She saw how she wouldn't manifest a job until she finished feeling all those unresolved emotions that created this belief. It wasn't until a year later that Naomi manifested a job that paid her enough so she could leave home. By this time, she had resolved many of those old issues and her relationship with her father was much better.

2. **What are your beliefs about money?** What beliefs did you grow up with? Go back to the beginning of the chapter and read the beliefs listed. Do they trigger any beliefs or memories in you? List the beliefs you remember. See how they relate to how much money you have in your life now.

For example, George worked as a plumbing contractor. His business was holding its own. Several times he attracted jobs that could make him a lot of money, but they all seemed to fall through at the last minute. It wasn't until George looked into his past that he discovered the belief that was creating this situation. Everyone loved his Uncle Rudy because he was happy, generous, and successful. He was also a gambler and extremely lucky. So when Uncle Rudy died in a car accident outside Las Vegas when George was seven, everyone in his family was very distraught, including George, who felt close to him. To this day, George can still remember his mother telling him how having too much money is bad for you. She claimed that's what killed Uncle Rudy. George took his mother's words to heart and began living that belief. He didn't want to make a lot of money, because he believed money killed you. It wasn't until George allowed himself to feel his fears and fully mourn his uncle's death that he was able to change this belief.

3. **What did your parents show you about money while you were growing up?** Did your parents believe that you had to save for a rainy day? Did they hoard, spend freely, recklessly? How important was money? How often did they talk about it? When they talked about it, how did they refer to it—that there was never enough, that it was bad for you or because of religious overtones, that it was evil? Did your parents try to control or manipulate you with it? How did their actions about money affect you? Are you just like them or do you polarize what they did?

For example, Stewart's father was a very successful man. Because he worked so hard and put in such long days, he spent little time with his son. Stewart felt that his mother really raised him. Yet Stewart never complained about his father's absences. After all, he was a good provider, and was always showing Stewart his love by buying him the things he wanted. When Stewart grew up and became a father, all the buried emotions of feeling ignored by his own father began to surface. They manifested in his life by having a job that didn't pay enough to make ends meet. Stewart worked a normal day. He had much more time to spend with his son than his father ever did with him. But he didn't have the money to provide for his son the way his father provided for him. In talking to Stewart, he realized several things. He realized that because of his father, he learned that the only way to make enough money was to work hard and long hours. He also learned that if you work that way, you miss out on your child's life. Stewart saw how he was hurt by his father's work ethic. He didn't want to be like his father and miss out on his own child's life. Once Stewart felt his hurt about his father, he was able to change his belief about making enough money.

4. **Did your parents use money to demonstrate their love because they didn't know any other way?** Do you have negative feelings about money because of this?

Gloria remembers her father as a good, quiet man. He worked hard, but never said much. Growing up, if she had a problem, she would look to her mother or friends for support. She couldn't talk to her father about anything. Yet she felt her father loved her. He lavished money on her and would take her shopping to the mall to buy her whatever she wanted. Gloria was married a year before she began having marital problems. She claimed her husband didn't love her. They always seemed to fight about money; especially when she wanted him to buy her something and he would refuse. It wasn't until Gloria felt the emotion of rejection, that she realized the problem. Her father taught her that money meant love. After all that was how he loved her: through money. When her husband failed to love her in the same manner, Gloria felt unloved. It wasn't until Gloria felt the emotions of being loved this way that she was able to change her definition of what love means.

5. **Do you feel like you will never have enough?** Having the feeling of not having enough comes from the feeling of not having your needs met when you were a baby. Go back to the first year of your life and try to discover how your needs weren't met. Look at your life now and compare to see if you are still living this pattern.

For example, when Mary Ann thinks about money, she thinks she will never have enough. Feeling this way doesn't make sense to her, because she grew up comfortably and still lives that way, even though now she is married and has two children. Yet the feeling surfaces every time she thinks about something she wants, but doesn't have. Like the new sofa for her living room, or the new wristwatch. She feels she will never have enough money to buy all the things she wants. When I asked Mary Ann what happened to her in the first year of her life, all she could remember was what her parents told her: that they moved into their new home when she was two weeks old. Her mother always described the experience as difficult. Mary Ann's delivery was by Caesarian, so her mother didn't have the energy to unpack, put everything away, and still watch and care for Mary Ann. Mary Ann never gave the move a second thought. Not until we began discussing it, did she realize that from a baby's point of view, the experience must have been scary, creating a tremendous sense of insecurity to a baby who didn't understand what was happening. Mary Ann clearly saw how her mother failed to give her the attention or the care she needed. She wasn't fed on time, or held, or responded to when she cried. To this day, Mary Ann was still reliving that experience of insecurity through her feelings about money and having things.

6. **How pragmatic are you? Do you believe that money is the only way to get what you want?** Do you believe in magic, miracles, or the power of 'mind over matter?' Or is money is the only realistic approach to getting what you want?

For example, take the case of two brothers. John is thirty-three and still believes in Santa Claus. He's a hopeless romantic who believes a guardian angel watches over him and takes good care of him. That's how he explains certain events in his life. Like the time he purchased a new home and the developer made an error and quoted him the wrong price, saving John twenty thousand dollars. Or the time he bought an old battered sofa from a garage sale for fifty dollars and later found five hundred stuffed in its lining.

His brother Carl thinks John is foolish and lives with his head in the clouds. Carl works for a bank and knows the value of money, how to invest it and make it work for you. Carl has never had any unusual experiences with money. After all, he's a realist and doesn't expect any.

7. **What is your attitude about getting things for free?** When someone gives you something for nothing, how do you feel? How easily do you accept it? What is your attitude about charity and being on the receiving end of it?

Take the case of Brad. Brad works very hard and lives from paycheck to paycheck. Brad is a proud, honest man, and well liked by the people in his community. He is always doing things to help others. People see how he struggles and want to help him in return. They offer to buy him the things he needs; yet Brad is too proud and refuses their offers.

8. **How much time during the day do you think about money?** Take the time to observe your thoughts. First of all, how much time do you spend thinking about money? Do you spend an inordinate amount of time? How are you thinking about it? Are your thoughts positive or negative? What is the emotion you feel when you think about money? Do you allow yourself to feel the emotion, or do you brush it aside in order to concentrate on what you need to do instead?

16

Using the Energy of Your Body to Heal Yourself

Just as you use your energy system to manifest what you want, you can also use your energy system to heal your body. In this chapter, I am going to explain once again several of the fundamental principles of the energy system of your body based on the System For Soul Memory that applies to healing. Let's reiterate what we know.

The Principles of the Body's Energy System According to the System for Soul Memory

1. Behind every injury or illness is an unresolved emotion.
2. Every injury or illness begins in the first eight years of life when the emotion first gets introduced then repressed.
3. All emotions reside in the chakras, the main energy centers of the body.
4. There are two ways the energy of an emotion can be released from the energy system of the body. The first way is by feeling the emotion as energy. The second way is by repressing the emotion until it becomes a physical malady in the body. At which time the energy of the emotion gets released as matter through the site of an injury or illness.

5. You must use the principle of transcendence in order to move energy and heal yourself. The principle of transcendence relies on using the combination of the physical, the emotional and the mental in order to gain wisdom and realize a result on the subatomic level of the soul. In using the principle of transcendence in healing, how, where, and the manner in which you get injured or sick, is considered the physical aspect. When you get sick or injured, strong emotions are released. Feeling these emotions is the emotional aspect. And finally, being aware of this entire healing process: knowing how you got sick, why you got sick, and naming the emotion that is making you sick, satisfies the mental requirements.

Once again, the System For Soul Memory believes that emotion drives energy. It triggers the thoughts that create the experiences. Every experience has an emotion behind it, driving it. Every experience is created by the soul to get you to 'know' this emotion transcendently. It wants you to 'know' it emotionally, physically, and mentally. All emotions are stored in the energy field of the body, more specifically in the chakras, the main energy centers. The soul has the job of keeping track of these emotions. It attracts the necessary people and events into your life to create the experiences that bring these emotions to the forefront. There are two ways the energy of an emotion can be felt. Either it is felt as pure energy. Or it is felt physically through the body as illness or injury. If the emotion was not felt at the time of its first introduction, then it is stored in the chakras where it is later recycled. You have seven years to feel the emotion once the soul presents it to you. If you do not feel it then, the next time the soul recycles the emotion, the experience will be more dramatic and severe. The longer an emotion sits in the chakra, the more compacted and denser the energy gets. Eventually the energy of the emotion becomes matter. As matter it travels first to the glands, then the organs of the body, then later, to other body parts. The chakra, where the emotion sits, will determine how and where the repressed energy will manifest physically in the body. Chapters 5 – 12 will tell you more.

Every injury or illness begins in the first eight years of life when the soul first introduces an emotion through the chakras. That is when every emotion you will ever know is introduced. On a more physical level, your DNA, or what you are born with, is a roadmap of those emotions you are here to know. To get a good idea of what experiences or illnesses you will create in your life, look at your ancestors. Their situations and illnesses will show you what your family did with their energy. You will probably do the same with yours. In other words, if diabetes runs in your family, then your family didn't know what to do the emotion of hopelessness. Maybe they acted it out by always partying, drinking, or doing something to help them forget the feeling. Or maybe they worked harder at proving that things weren't so hopeless. Or maybe they just ignored the feeling. Whatever they did, if they suffered from diabetes, they did not feel the emotion.

The Healing Process

According to the System For Soul Memory, the soul gives you two ways to experience an emotion. You can either feel the emotion as energy, or you can experience the emotion as physical matter. In other words, the longer the emotion sits in the energy field the more compacted it gets until it finally becomes physical matter. When this happens, you experience the emotion as a physical injury or illness.

Once an emotion becomes a physical malady in the body, there are two ways to heal. The first way is to feel the emotion as energy. When the emotion is felt and released as energy, the compacted matter of the malady gets broken down and reabsorbed into the body, allowing the body to heal. The second way is to physically remove the diseased or injured part of the body. This method has its drawbacks. It only works if you can afford to lose a body part like a finger, a limb, or an organ that is not life sustaining. Also, removing the body part sometimes only removes part of the unprocessed emotion. One emotion can have several other emotions attached to it. You will know this to be the case, when you continue to experience health problems even after the diseased body part is removed.

The soul doesn't want you to lose a body part. The soul would rather you heal by *feeling* the repressed emotion. Throughout the healing process, the soul gives you repeated chances to feel the emotion again by creating new events to trigger the release of the buried emotion. At any stage of the healing process, when a buried emotion is felt as emotional energy, healing occurs. The quicker you feel the emotion, the quicker you heal. If you are slow to feel the emotion, your healing process will be slow and drawn out.

If you remain steadfast in not dealing with the emotion, if you continue to manipulate and stifle the flow of energy to the point where the body can no longer survive, you leave the soul no choice but to leave the body. In other words, you die.

Helping Yourself to Heal

Through the years, I discovered many people have a hard time accepting responsibility for their illness or injury. They don't want to go deeper and accept that an emotion caused their problem. Most people would rather give their healing responsibilities to their doctors. They would rather sit back and wait for medicine to cure them. I found that doing both works very well. When you tell your soul you are willing to work on the emotion causing your illness or injury and begin to feel it, your soul will attract the right doctors, medical procedures, and medicines to help you heal.

For example, Tamara was a customer of my bookstore. She was only 28 years old, yet she was slowly going blind. There was nothing the doctors could do for her. As her eyesight worsened, Tamara came into the store looking for alternative methods to see if she could heal herself. Tamara began to meditate and used various breathing techniques. Slowly her life began to change as she focused inwardly and started learning about herself. Quite often, when she came into the store to tell me about events that were happening, I would show her how to stay centered and feel the emotions they triggered. One day Tamara came in and told me she was moving to South Africa. She felt a strong pull to go there. Three months later, Tamara wrote me a letter. While in South Africa, she heard about a doctor with a new surgical technique that could cure her eye problem. I knew Tamara was ready to heal. She did her work by feeling many of the buried emotions causing her eye problem. Now her soul was putting her on the final journey by attracting the means for a quick recovery.

If you want to use the energy system of your body to heal yourself, there are several things you must do.

1. *You must accept your illness or injury.*

You must accept that you are the creator of your illness or injury. When you claim your power in creating your illness or injury, you claim your power to heal it. You acknowledge that your soul created the situation. Only by aligning yourself with your soul will you find the necessary abilities to heal.

When you accept and validate your illness or injury, you must also be willing to accept everything about it. You must be willing to accept that on some level, you wanted to physically hurt yourself. Once you accept this, strong feelings of sadness emerge. These feelings originate from all the times you fought yourself, ignored yourself, and denied processing your own emotions. You demonstrated to your soul how you felt about yourself, that you don't love or accept a part of yourself. Opening yourself to these emotions allows the healing process to begin.

Also, if you create a life-threatening injury or illness, you must accept that a part of you wants to die. You must examine your life and find out why. You must feel the emotions and the desire that is making you want to die. People are always horrified when I tell them this. They say to me, "If I feel the emotion of wanting to die,

I will surely die." I always point out to these people that they are already *living* the emotion of wanting to die. *Feeling* the emotion frees the blocked energy that is creating the life-threatening situation. Freeing the blocked energy creates life and allows the healing to begin. If you are *living* the experience of being sick or injured to the point where your life is threatened, then you are not *feeling* the emotion of wanting to die.

The feeling of wanting to die is a normal emotion for many children. A child not getting his or her way or feeling abused and helpless, may, in a moment, feel the desire to die. A near death incident in childhood like almost drowning, or being in a car accident would also trigger the feeling of dying, and could be the seed pattern for the emotion in adulthood. Look back to your childhood and see if you can remember a time that was so depressing, or an incident that almost took your life, to discover where this emotion first originated.

2. *You must take responsibility for your injury or illness.*

You must take full responsibility for what you created in your life. You can't be a victim. If you believe that you are sick or injured because of what someone or something did to you, you will never fully heal. In other words, if you think you got lung cancer from smoking cigarettes, or if you think you got heart disease because of high cholesterol, which runs in the family, then you will never heal. You cannot be a victim if you want to heal. In order to use the energy system of your body to heal, you must take full responsibility for your illness or injury. You must accept that your soul created your injury or illness to get you to deal with an emotion you have been avoiding since childhood. Your soul got you to smoke or eat foods high in cholesterol. Your soul attracted them into your life because of an emotion you were avoiding. Your constant denial, in dealing with this emotion, forced your soul to take desperate actions.

You also can't sit back and let others make your healing decisions for you. If you want to heal, you must be the main participant in your healing process. You must make the decisions in how you want to be treated. You must be positive you want to heal. Being sick or injured has its good points besides the obvious bad points. Generally when you are sick or injured, you are receiving more attention than usual. You are receiving more care and love. Being well means you will have to give this up. If you are having trouble healing, this may be one of the reasons why. If this is the case, then one of the emotions you are not feeling is the emotion of loneliness, or feeling unloved.

3. *You must use the principles of transcendence in order to heal.*

Healing can only occur when body, mind and soul are actively used in the healing process. Soul represents the emotional aspect. In order to heal, you must feel the emotions causing your illness or injury. The body represents all physical aspects of your injury or illness. In order to heal, you must be aware of where you are sick or injured the physical circumstances in how you got that way, and how you are physically being treated. And third, the mental represents your thoughts and intentions during the healing process. In order to heal, you must stay focused inwardly and be aware of what is going on inside you as well as outside you.

In meditation, when you are in a transcendent state, your brain waves are in the delta-state. Delta is the deepest sleep-state of the brain. This is the state where healing occurs in the body. The longer you stay in a delta-state, the more time you give your body to heal. In other words, the more time you spend in transcendence, in the awareness of how you think and feel, emotionally and physically, the more time you give your body to heal itself.

4. *You must use emotion to move energy to heal.*

You must feel the repressed emotion causing your injury or illness if you want to heal. Besides feeling this emotion, you can also use an energy stimulator to quicken the healing process. In Chapter 14, I discuss the use of three energy stimulators that are more potent in getting energy moving. They are will, desire, and anger. Any three will work in getting the compacted emotional energy moving so you can feel it and heal. When you use an energy stimulator you are creating the *intention* to heal. This would be no different than praying, using creative visualization, or saying affirmations. You are focusing your desire and will to manifest what you want.

At this point I wish to mention the difference between intention and attitude. Countless times I have been in the presence of someone who is very ill, and had a good attitude. Yet, I knew their good attitude was killing them. It was preventing them from feeling all the emotions the soul was trying to get them to feel to heal. Having a good attitude can be detrimental if it keeps you from feeling your emotions. It can mask many feelings. When you are sick or injured, you want to feel depressed, sad, helpless, angry, grumpy, or mean. You want to feel everything. You don't want to mask all those feelings behind the façade of having a good attitude. Also, having the façade of a good attitude can mask hidden hurts from your childhood. When you were young, did your parents expect you to have a good attitude? What happened if your attitude wasn't good? Were you punished, rejected, sent to your room?

When you are sick or injured, you want to have *strong intentions*, not necessarily a good attitude. You want to take your ability to create, and use it to manifest good health. You want to use your will power, your desire, and your anger to change your life and the state of your health. You want to take this time to concentrate solely on yourself. You want please yourself as much as you can, instead of trying to please or placate others. Your soul has created this difficult time to force you to look at yourself. In order to heal, you must use the time and do it.

5. *You must allow for any changes healing will create in your life.*

When you begin to feel the emotions causing your malady, your life will begin to change. In order to heal, you must allow for the changes. Before your injury or illness, something in your life wasn't working right. It was causing you stress. In order to heal, you must be willing to assess whatever it was, and let it go. You must be willing to make changes. In making the changes, you are telling your soul you are willing to accept good health.

How to Find the Buried Emotion Causing Your Injury or Illness

If at this moment you are sick or suffering with an injury, then you are not feeling an emotion that has been suppressed since childhood. If you can discover what that emotion is, and feel it, you will speed your healing process.

If you are sick or injured and have no clue what emotion is triggering your situation, there are several things you can do to help you uncover it.

1. What happened to you just before you injured yourself?

Think back to the incidents proceeding your injury. There is usually one particular incident that triggered a strong emotion. When you didn't feel the emotion as energy, the soul created the injury to get you to feel it.

For example, Cathy got into a major disagreement with her friend Cheryl. Cheryl didn't see or speak to Cathy again. A year later, Cathy saw Cheryl in the grocery store. Cathy said hello, but Cheryl walked by her. This brought up all the old emotions Cathy had originally avoided. The next day, Cathy was late to work. She was running from her car to the office, when she slipped and fell in the parking lot. Cathy hurt her back. When Cathy was asked to review the emotions she experienced in the parking lot, she listed several. She felt angry that she fell. She felt helpless that she couldn't walk and had to wait for someone to call for help. And last, she felt like she did something wrong, because if she hadn't been late and running, she wouldn't have injured herself. After further contemplation, Cathy realized these emotions were similar to what she felt seeing Cheryl again. She was *angry,* that even after a year, Cheryl was still ignoring her. She *felt powerless* to the situation. She also felt, that in expressing her opinion, *she did something wrong*, which made Cheryl never want to speak to her again. After Cathy felt all the feelings, she remembered a similar incident occurring when she was five years old. She was in the grocery store with her mother. It was Halloween and she wanted to see the candy display, but her mother was in a hurry and wouldn't let her. Cathy threw a tantrum. She managed to escape her mother, only to run head long into the candy display, toppling it. Cathy's mother was so angry, she never let Cathy forget the incident.

Cathy healed quickly once she felt all the emotions and fulfilled the requirements of transcendence.

2. **If you are sick, think back several months to a year before your illness manifested, and search for any traumatic incidents.**

Chances are there was a traumatic incident that you never dealt with emotionally. This incident could have been physical like a change in life, losing your job, changing your job, moving, divorce, relationship problems, someone dying, or just being hit with something that upset you.

For example, Betsy's husband, Bernie, and his brother were in business together. When Bernie discovered that his brother was stealing from the business, Betsy's whole life changed. Her brother-in-law skipped town leaving them with large debts, angry suppliers, and a business worth nothing. Betsy and Bernie were forced to sell their home to pay the debt. They had to move to a new town so Bernie could find work. Three months after settling into their new apartment, Betsy got sick. The doctors found a tumor on her right kidney, which required surgery. In looking back, Betsy realized she felt victimized by her brother-in-law. Even worse, Betsy felt much bitterness towards Bernie for letting her down and not keeping her safe.

3. **Can you remember what emotion you felt when you first injured yourself?**

The minute your accident occurred and you realized you were injured, what did you feel? Did you allow yourself to feel the emotion, or did you suppress it?

Within the first hour of an injury, the strongest release of emotion is experienced through the site of the injury. If you are aware of the emotion at this time and feel it, your healing process will be quick and easy. When children are injured, they heal quickly. They heal quickly, because when they are injured, they immediately cry and express emotion. They don't hold anything back. You can heal just as quickly if you allow yourself to cry and feel your emotions the moment you are injured.

4. Can you remember what emotion you felt when you were first told you were sick?

Finding out that you are seriously ill can immediately put you into a state of shock. It may be days before your true emotions emerge. Think back to when you first got your news and remember how you reacted. Were you in a state of denial? Did you easily accept it? Were you in shock? Did you feel your emotions as they surfaced, or did you suppress them?

For example, Carl suffered a heart attack. The doctors told him he needed triple bypass surgery. Carl was always an energetic man. He loved to jog, stay out late, work hard. The doctor told him his life style was going to have to change. Carl wouldn't allow the doctor's prognosis to get him down. He was determined to live life the way he was accustomed. Unfortunately the doctor was right. Carl's body betrayed him. He couldn't do the things he normally did. Carl never felt the emotions this triggered. Especially the feeling of hopelessness that his body would never be the same again. A year later, Carl developed diabetes. This caused further complications in his healing process.

5. Think about your healing process. Were there any special events that occurred? Can you name the emotions they triggered in you?

Did anything unusual happen during your illness? For instance, did you have any complications? Did you have any reverse reactions to medication given you? Did something happen to make your illness more stressful, like health insurance problems, family problems?

The events that occur during your healing process are created by your soul to get you to feel an emotion you are still avoiding. As long as you avoid the emotion, you will remain sick. The soul wants you to heal. It repeatedly gives you new experiences to trigger the emotions to get you to heal. Your healing process is a map showing you which emotions you are avoiding.

For example, Ginger has breast cancer. After surgery, the doctors told her she needed chemotherapy. Ginger has two daughters and works full time running the office for her husband's drapery business. Ginger feels she doesn't have time to be sick. She has too many responsibilities, too much to do, and no family close enough to help her. Within weeks after the surgery, Ginger is back at work. Even with the chemotherapy, Ginger doesn't slow down. She stops her tears when she feels too sick, or so tired she can't move another muscle. She won't let herself think about her prognosis. Too many people are relying on her. Ginger develops a reaction to the chemotherapy. It severely affects her heart and forces her to be bedridden for several months. Her mother has to travel from a different state to take care of her. Her husband has to hire someone else to run his office. Ginger's soul managed very nicely to stop her life, force her to slow down and accept help, so that she would have enough time to deal with her emotions.

6. Are you still suffering with some aspect of your injury or illness? Are you still sore or tender? Because of it, do you have to make changes in your lifestyle?

Your soul is not going to let you go back to your normal lifestyle until you deal with the emotions you are still suppressing.

Think about any changes in lifestyle you are making. What emotions surface when you think about them? Are there any particular thoughts that keep hounding you? Do these emotions remind you of another time, another situation, or another person?

For example, Eric works for a meat packing company. In February, he slipped on some ice while shoveling his sidewalk and shattered his elbow. Eric's elbow never healed properly, forcing him to find new work. While searching for a new job, all Eric could think about was his old boss, and how he made Eric feel incompetent, that he wasn't good enough. Eric kept telling himself that he was happy to be finding new work. Now he wouldn't have to see his old boss again.

By forcing Eric to think about his old boss, his soul was trying to get Eric to feel the emotions of unworthiness and poor self-esteem still buried in the energy field around his elbow. If Eric felt those emotions, he would heal completely. If Eric didn't feel them, he would continue to have elbow problems. He would also attract a new boss who was just as abusive as the old one, continuing Eric's old pattern. The soul does what it must to get you to feel your emotions.

7. **Sometimes you sacrifice a part of your body to heal yourself of an emotion. If this happened to you, how did your life change after your sacrifice?**

For example, Joan was married to a man who cheated on her for years. Joan never confronted Arthur. She looked the other way, just as her mother did when her father did the same thing. Joan began suffering with female problems. She bled heavily during her periods and developed fibroid tumors. Then, one day, Joan's husband walked in and told her he was in love with another woman and wanted a divorce. After the divorce Joan's female problems got worse. The doctor told her she would need a hysterectomy. A year after the divorce, Joan met another man who was kind, faithful and nothing like her ex. Also at this time, Joan had her hysterectomy. If you asked Joan why she had the surgery, her response was "That was my way of getting rid of Arthur."

8. Which chakra is the source for your injury or illness?

If you are sick and injured and still have no clue what emotion you are repressing, reading Chapters 5-12, on the different chakras, should enable you to pinpoint the source chakra that is causing your injury or illness. Pinpointing the chakra will help you discover what emotion you are repressing. It will help you go back to your childhood and discover the seed pattern, where your hurt first started.

For example, Lisa has a brain tumor. Surgery goes well, and the doctors say the tumor is benign. Lisa is only thirty-three years old. She can't imagine why she got sick. When reading the chapters about the chakras, she realizes that both the Third Eye Chakra and the Crown Chakra deal with the brain. These chakras develop during the ages of seven and eight. Lisa remembers that her parents separated and got divorced when she was seven and eight years old. This gave Lisa a good idea which emotions she was repressing. In thinking about her life just prior to her illness, Lisa realized another factor that would have triggered her tumor. Six months before she got sick, her mother told her she was getting divorced again.

9. If you are sick, something in your life isn't working right. It is causing you stress. Can you pinpoint what it is?

What in your life do you hate, or that you wish you could change? Every hate, irritant, annoyance, or unwanted activity has an unfelt emotion behind it triggering it. Until you process that emotion, you will not be able to heal. Sometimes, making physical changes helps you to feel those emotions.

For example, Darren has prostate cancer. In thinking about what he hates about his life, Darren realizes that it is his lifestyle. He has everything. A big house, fancy sports car, anything he could want monetarily. But in order to maintain this lifestyle, he has to work eighty hours a week. He feels like a slave to his job and his possessions. After Darren gets out of the hospital, he quits his job, and puts his house on the market to sell. His wife thinks he is acting irrationally. Her reaction triggers strong emotions in him. These are the strong emotions that caused his cancer originally. By making drastic changes in his lifestyle, Darren was going to heal himself.

10. Every physical pain in the body is an unrealized emotion. If you had to guess, what emotion would you say is causing your pain? Is there a person in your life who aggravates you? Is there a situation that gives you grief? Figuring out what pains you in your life will help you figure out what emotion you are suppressing.

Don't discount the first thing that pops into your head when you answer the above questions. For instance, Jeremy got into a minor car accident. He experienced severe whiplash and was forced to wear a neck brace for several weeks. A year later he was still experiencing pain in his neck. One day, when he backed out from playing sports with his friends, he joked, "My girlfriend is giving me a pain in the neck." Everyone laughed because they knew Jeremy had a great relationship. His remark was the farthest thing from the truth.

On further inspection though, Jeremy's remark was right on target. Jeremy's girlfriend was nagging him about a particular subject that reminded him of the way his mother nagged him when he was a boy. This really irritated Jeremy, and brought up many old feelings. He was surprised that the pain in his neck was connected to the way his girl friend was treating him.

11. Go back seven to eight years. Can you remember something happening in your life that was traumatic or emotionally draining?

Emotions 'snowball' after every seven years. In other words, if you don't feel them when they are 'snowflakes', they will eventually become 'avalanches.' Generally you can follow the pattern of this happening in your life. If you can't remember a traumatic incident happening just before your injury or illness, go back to another seven-year cycle and see if you can remember something traumatic happening then.

For example, Marlene is twenty-six and trying to get pregnant. The doctor told her that because of fibroid tumors in her uterus, she was going to have problems. So far, medication and minor surgical procedures weren't helping. Marlene couldn't think of anything in her current life that would cause this problem. Yet going back to another seven-year cycle, Marlene thought about her teenage years. Immediately, she knew the traumatic event causing her inability to get pregnant. When she was in high school, she was date raped by one of her classmates. They were fooling around in a car, when he became insensitive to her pleas to stop.

Marlene immediately realized the connection to her life now. Her husband was being just as insensitive to her plight about getting pregnant.

12. Why do you think you wanted to hurt yourself? Or why do you think you wanted to be sick?

Don't think about your answer. Allow it to come spontaneously, no matter how outrageous it seems. Your soul will give you clues in the answer.

For example, Jason was home from college for Christmas break. He and some friends decided to go skiing. He was fooling around with his friends, experimenting with snowboarding, when he fell and severely damaged his knee. He required surgery and months of physical therapy before he could walk normally again. He missed a semester from school. If you asked Jason why he hurt himself, his answer was, "I was so tired, I just wanted a month in bed."

During Jason's convalescence, he realized that he wasn't happy at college; that he was involved in too many activities with a fraternity that was making him miserable. At the time he didn't realize it. Being in bed for a month gave him plenty of time to feel his emotions and evaluate his situation.

Cancer

The emotion that causes cancer is hate. Love keeps the cells of your body happy and functioning normally. Hate makes the cells go out of control. If you suffer with cancer, there is something, someone or some aspect of your life that you hate. You are not allowing yourself to feel the emotion, or resolve the circumstances causing your hate. Hate begins in the first eight years of life when the soul presents your learning lessons to you. If you suffer from cancer, then hate is one of the emotions you are here to learn. Hate is the polarity of love. Without hate, you won't know love. If you think of hate in religious terms as being bad and should be avoided, you will have trouble feeling the emotion. If you think of hate as being just another emotion, you will feel it easily.

If you have cancer, you have repressed your hate to the point where you are willing to die. Suffering with cancer is very grave. On the level of the soul, you are choosing life or death. Only when you allow yourself to feel your hate will you choose life.

If you have trouble discerning what you hate, where your cancer sits in your body, will give you a clue which chakra is involved. Within this chakra sits your hate. I will give you some examples.

The Root Chakra—if you suffer from prostate cancer, bladder cancer, testicular cancer, or rectal cancer, your hate is manifesting in the Root Chakra. The Root Chakra develops from the time of conception through the first year of life. Did any event occur to you during this time that you think about and hate? Also, the Root Chakra deals with issues concerning the father, where you live, how you live, work, career, and environment. Examine your life in these areas to discover what you hate. There could be some aspect of your father that really irritates you. You could feel so insecure in the area where you live, that you hate it. You could be so disappointed in your career, that you hate working.

The Navel Chakra—if you suffer from colon cancer, kidney cancer, breast cancer, cervical cancer, or uterine cancer, your hate sits in the Navel Chakra. The Navel Chakra develops through the age of two. Did any event occur to you during this time that you think about and hate? This chakra also deals with issues concerning the mother, feeling victimized, feeling unsupported, and feelings of self-sacrifice and martyrdom. Examine your life in these areas to discover what you hate. There could be some aspect of your mother that really irritates you. Maybe you are feeling victimized by someone or something and you hate it. Maybe you hate that you are not getting enough support from your loved ones. Or maybe you hate the fact that you made a sacrifice that you later regretted.

The Solar Plexus Chakra—if you suffer from stomach cancer, liver cancer, or pancreatic cancer, your hate is manifesting in the Solar Plexus Chakra. The Solar Plexus Chakra develops through the age of three. Did any event occur to you during this time that you think about and hate? This chakra also deals with issues of feeling powerless, and hopeless. It is also the seat of your anger. Examine your life in these areas to discover what you hate. There could be something that makes you feel so powerless you hate yourself. Or maybe you hate what makes you feel so powerless. Maybe you feel you are always struggling and hate that you are going nowhere. Or maybe you hate your anger. Do you have an issue with violence? Do you hate your parents for the times when they released their anger on you?

The Heart Chakra—if you suffer from lung cancer, or cancer in the Thymus Gland or in tissues around the heart, your hate sits in the Heart Chakra. The Heart Chakra develops through the age of four. Did any event occur to you during this time that you think about and hate? Also, this chakra deals with issues concerning love, rejection and betrayal. Examine your life in these areas to discover what you hate. There could be someone who betrayed you that you hate. Or maybe you hate yourself for betraying someone you love. Maybe you hate someone for rejecting you. Or vice verse, you rejected someone and you hate yourself for it.

The Throat Chakra—if you suffer from throat cancer, mouth cancer, cancer of the esophagus, cancer of the larynx, or thyroid cancer, your hate sits in the Throat Chakra. The Throat Chakra develops through the age of five. Did any event occur to you during this time that you think about and hate? Also, this chakra deals with how you relate to the people closest to you and how they relate to you. Your feelings of self-esteem begin in this chakra. Examine your life in these areas to discover what you hate. There could be someone you hate because they are constantly criticizing you or putting you down. Maybe you hate yourself for something you once said. Do you hate how you feel about yourself? Maybe you hate that you are not good enough. Or maybe you hate that someone you love thinks you are not good enough. Do you hate that your talents are not accepted, or wasted? Do you hate yourself for not speaking up for yourself?

The Moon Center Chakra—if you suffer from bone cancer, leukemia, AIDs, skin cancer, or cancer of the Hypothalamus gland, your hate sits in the Moon Center Chakra. The Moon Center Chakra develops through the age of six. Did any event occur to you during this time that you think about and hate? Also, this chakra deals with how you relate to the outside world. Just as in the Throat Chakra, your feelings of self-esteem are also tied into this chakra. Examine your life in these areas to discover what you hate. Do you hate that you feel different, that you feel like you don't fit in? Do you hate someone in your life because he or she is constantly shaming you, or they shamed you in the past? Maybe you hate someone who is constantly judging you. Do you hate yourself for being too hard on yourself? Do you hate all the responsibilities foisted on you? Do you hate living? Do you hate yourself for something you did in the past?

The Third Eye Chakra—if you suffer from brain cancer, cancer of the Pituitary gland, or cancer of the eye, your cancer sits in the Third Eye Chakra. The Third Eye Chakra develops through the age of seven. Did any event occur to you during this time that you think about and hate? Also, this chakra deals with your beliefs and how they are accepted. Examine your life in this area to discover what you hate. There could be someone you hate who is constantly rejecting your beliefs. Maybe you hate someone for his or her beliefs. Do you hate someone for forcing his or her beliefs or will on you? Or do you hate yourself for forcing your beliefs or will on someone else? Maybe you hate the church, or your religion, or God, because of something that was done to you in the name of religion. Maybe you hate yourself because someone was hurt because of your beliefs. You could also hate yourself because you were hurt or disappointed by your own beliefs. Did someone with mental problems mistreat you and do you hate them because of it? Did this cause you to fear yourself and hate any mental instability within you?

The Crown Chakra—if you suffer from brain cancer or cancer of the Pineal gland, your hate sits in the Crown Chakra. The Crown Chakra develops through the age of eight. Did any event occur to you during this time that you think about and hate? Also, this chakra deals with how you accept yourself or how others accept you. Examine your life in this area to discover what you hate. Does your hate manifest because you can't accept yourself or someone else? Is your hate directed inward because you can't accept your life? Do you hate your thoughts and feelings so much that you put your brain on overload trying to control them? Do you hate how emotional you are? Do you hate yourself? Is there someone you hate because they never accepted you?

Insights on Different Illnesses

Below is a listing of some of the illnesses I have encountered. Being in the energy fields of those who suffer from these diseases allowed me to feel the emotions that were being suppressed. Most diseases are a combination of emotional blocks found in several chakras. Sometimes in trying to control, or suppress one emotion, another emotion from another chakra is used to mask it or manipulate it. How you manipulate your energy and your blocked emotions, cause a particular disease to manifest.

A. **Multiple Sclerosis:** There are two overpowering emotions that cause this disease. The first emotion is shame. Shame is found in the Moon Center Chakra which controls the muscles of the body and how much movement you have. The second emotion is feeling powerless. This emotion is found in the Solar Plexus Chakra, which controls how much energy you have. What creates this particular disease is the manipulation of a third emotion, that of pride, to mask the emotions of shame and powerlessness. Pride is found in the Third Eye Chakra, which controls the central nervous system. The willful use of pride to stifle the energy of shame, and of feeling powerless, causes the breakdown of the nerve endings in the brain. The body slowly becomes paralyzed and helpless.

B. **Asthma:** asthma in children generally means that a parent is not allowing the child's true nature to be good enough. They are smothering the child with too many 'should and shouldn'ts', trying to make the child better. For instance, if a child's true nature is to be a dreamer, causing the child to daydream in class or suffer in school, a parent might force the child to be more grounded. This creates stress for the child to be something he or she isn't. Generally the child outgrows the asthma, as he or she become an adult. Once a child is away from the smothering attitude of the parent, he or she gains the freedom to be who they truly are. If as an adult they are still suffering from the asthma, then they are still not allowing their true nature to emerge. Asthma is found in the Moon Center Chakra, where in the medulla oblongata, the breathing control center is found.

C. **Thyroid problems:** Having thyroid problems means you are getting criticized too much. Your self-esteem is low and you don't feel good enough about yourself. What happened to you at the age of five? Who in your family made you feel this way? Who's criticizing you today? Or are you acting out your feelings by criticizing others? The thyroid is found in the Throat Chakra.

D. **AIDs:** Shame and feeling different are the two emotions that help to create this disease. These emotions do not only belong to gay people. These emotions are found in the Moon Center Chakra, home of the Hypothalamus Gland. This disease involves the immune system, which means the person suffering with the disease feels like he or she is being attacked for feeling different.

E. **Crohns or Colitis:** This disease resides mainly in the Navel Chakra. The emotion is feeling unsafe and violated in your surrounding. I discovered that what usually causes this feeling is a strong or overbearing parent. Because the parent's actions come from a place of love, the sensitive child learns to bury the feeling of aggressiveness. The aura of a person suffering with this condition is a muddied yellow, the same color of someone suffering with a virus or bacterial disease. Therefore the Moon Center Chakra, the director of the immune system is involved. Again, whenever the immune system is involved, there is a feeling of being invaded or attacked.

F. **Addison's Disease:** This is a disease of the Adrenal Gland found in the Navel Chakra. Again this disease is based in childhood. The emotions are those of bitterness and resentment towards a parent who is needy, and too overprotective. The child has been made to feel they are his or her parent's sole reason for living, or that the parent sacrifices their life for them. This puts tremendous stress on the child. But because the love between parent and child is strong, the child feels guilty for feeling this way and learns to bury his or her resentment and bitterness.

G. **Diabetes:** The emotion that causes this disease is hopelessness. It is generally found in people as they get older when they discover life has disappointed them. If a child is born with this disease, then look at the genetic patterning of the family. The feeling of hopelessness will be a strong influence through the generations. This disease is found in the Solar Plexus Chakra.

H. **Prostate problems or cancer:** The men I've encountered with this condition are men who are pressured by their careers or worry about how they are going to pay their bills. It is a work-related issue where their very sense of manliness is dependent on how well they earn. These issues begin in childhood with their relationship with the father. If there is prostate cancer, then look back to see if there is any hate for the father. The prostate is found in the Root Chakra.

I. **Heart problems:** Most problems dealing with the heart such as heart attack, hardening of the arteries, and cholesterol problems, are linked to old issues of abandonment. The heart is found in the Heart Chakra.

J. **Arthritis:** Arthritis is found in the Moon Center Chakra, which controls the joints of the body. People who suffer from arthritis feel unappreciated. They are people who do things for others, but are not acknowledged for the things they do. Sometimes the things they do meets with resistance. For instance, maybe these people do volunteer work or work with charities and their work goes unappreciated. Or maybe these people do things for their family that goes unnoticed. Or maybe they are working for a business or an organization where there are too many obstacles in what they are trying to achieve.

K. **Breast Cancer:** Women who suffer with breast cancer don't know how to be nurtured or supported. These are usually the women who are super-moms, or strongly independent. They don't know how to ask for help, nor do they usually get it. They were taught early by their mothers not to expect it. Breast cancer is caused by unresolved feelings of hate for the mother. It could be one particular thing the mother said or did, or a part of the mother's personality that is annoying or stressful.

L. **Tonsillitis:** This usually occurs within six months after a highly emotional, stressful situation. An event occurred where feelings were hurt, but not voiced. Therefore, all those emotions that weren't expressed are creating blocked energy, which is irritating the throat. The tonsils are found in the Throat Chakra.

M. **Allergies:** Being allergic to something means you feel powerless to it. If an incident occurs which is emotionally traumatic, you will feel vulnerable and powerless to everything involved in that incident. This includes the environment, what you were doing or what you were eating. If you were eating chicken when your lover told you he was leaving, you could develop an allergy to chicken. If, when you were five and you were outside climbing trees with your friends and your mother yelled at you, humiliating you in front of them, you could develop an allergy to tree pollen. If you suffer from an allergy take the object you are allergic to and see if you can remember a traumatic incident which included it. Feeling the emotion of the traumatic incident will heal the allergy.

N. **Problems with the teeth or gums:** If you suffer with poor teeth or gums, then you are not feeling the emotion of shame. The teeth are part of the Moon Center Chakra. Look back to your childhood and try to remember an incident that made you feel ashamed. Maybe there was a person who made you feel this way. Even though the Moon Center Chakra develops during the age of six, the incident did not necessarily have to take place then. This emotion can be attached to other emotions found in different chakras. Next time you have a tooth or gum problem, look back to the previous few months. Did any incidents occur where you felt shamed? If you feel your shame, you will prevent further problems with your teeth.

O. **Colds:** When you are feeling overwhelmed by events in your life, when you have too much happening at once, you will catch a cold. It is the soul's way of slowing you down so you can process all the emotions hitting you at once. Colds are a virus, and any time you catch a virus, you feel you are being attacked. This feeling engages the immune system to respond. The immune system is found in the Moon Center Chakra.

P. **Flu, stomach virus, or other viruses:** If you are suffering with a virus, once again, because it involves the immune system and the Moon Center Chakra, you are feeling attacked. Look back to the last few weeks and examine your life. Did anybody come down hard on you? Did they force their opinion on you? Did you feel threatened in any way? Did any event occur where you felt attacked? Were you overly emotional and felt threatened by your emotions?

Q. **Minor cuts, scrapes or injuries:** if you cut yourself, burned yourself or injured yourself in any minor way, you were not processing an emotion that occurred just before your injury. Think back to what you were feeling just before you hurt yourself, to discover what it is.

R. **Gallstones:** If you suffer with gallstones, then you are feeling stymied. You are having trouble making decisions. You are feeling powerless that you don't know what to do. You are either acting out this feeling or you are judging yourself for being this way. Either way, you are not allowing yourself to feel the emotion. Gallstones are found in the Solar Plexus Chakra.

S. **Hemorrhoids:** If you suffer with hemorrhoids, you are worried about what you are doing with your life. It is the feeling that what you are doing has no value. You are feeling worthless. This will manifest in the area of your career. You may feel like you are wasting your time, or that you are not being constructive. Hemorrhoids are found in the Root Chakra.

17

Most Frequently Asked Questions About the System for Soul Memory

When people begin using the System For Soul Memory, there are several questions often asked. Below is a listing of those questions.

1. How do I know when I have finished feeling an emotion?

When you are no longer *living* the emotion, you know you have finished feeling it. For example: When you have finished feeling the emotion of loneliness, you will no longer be lonely. You will feel better about yourself and will begin attracting new people into your life. When you have finished feeling the emotion of feeling impoverished, you will no longer have money problems. You will begin attracting money, or new earning situations that will bring you more abundance. When you have finished feeling the emotion of craving love through negative means, you will no longer be abused. In other words, your life will reflect whether or not you have finished feeling the emotion.

Also, if you have strong feelings of animosity towards someone, these feelings will disappear when you have finished feeling the emotions concerning them. Incredibly, you will feel compassion instead. This is another indication that you have finished feeling an emotion.

Some emotions are so deep and painful they take several years and several stages to work through. You may feel an emotion, have it leave your life, then re-experience it again several years later. The soul knows how much you can handle, so it presents the emotion to you in stages so you can deal with it better.

2. How am I supposed to feel an emotion when I am working, or in a crowd full of people?

If you are unable to feel your emotions when they occur because you are at work, or because you are too busy reacting to the situation, then you can still feel them later when you are home or alone. All you have to do is be aware of the emotion that is surfacing at the time of the incident and flag it with the thought that you will feel it later. Generally, you have a couple of days to feel the emotion. It will be strongest in the beginning. Then it will slowly dissipate. During this time, just focussing your attention back on the emotion will bring it to the surface again.

3. If I start crying, I will cry forever. What should I do?

If someone is working on a really deep issue from their childhood, it could take months, or even a year to work through the various emotions attached to it. That's why people complain to me that all they do is cry. Yet if you think about it logically, you will gain a better understanding of the process. Usually these people had a miserable childhood. They lived under painful conditions for many years. Within their chakras, they buried years worth of hurt. Once they allowed the old hurt to come forth, they began the process of release, crying for the many years of pain. Therefore, it is not logical to expect years worth of pain to take only several days' worth of crying to remedy. When people tell me they feel like they will cry forever, they are telling me their pain is deep. A few *months* of crying, is really in effect, the *years* worth of crying they never allowed in the past.

Therefore, if you feel like you will cry forever, you won't. You are only crying for the feelings you already know about, those feelings you have been carrying around since childhood. Continue to feel all the emotions that come up. Your soul won't give you more than you can handle.

Feeling like you will cry forever is actually another emotion to be felt. It could be the emotion of feeling helpless or hopeless when you were younger. By concentrating on the feeling, you will eventually know which emotion it is. By feeling it, you will gain the wisdom and go beyond it.

Through the years I discovered that some people cry without feeling an emotion. These people are more caught up in the act of crying, than in feeling the emotion behind it. Therefore, be sure you are feeling your emotions when you cry. Otherwise, crying becomes like a defense drama, a physical act that buries an emotion instead of releasing it.

4. I thought I felt the emotions before, why am I feeling them again?

Sometimes when an emotion is very deep and painful, the soul will release it in stages. This is done to protect you. The soul knows how much you can handle. When this happens, you will feel the emotion little by little over a period of months or years. The first time you feel it, it will be very difficult to feel. Yet each time subsequently, it will be easier, even though you will be getting deeper into the hurt. By the time you get to the bottom of it, you will be in total awareness of the hurt. You will know the procedure of releasing it and won't feel so overwhelmed by it.

5. I've been feeling so many emotions I can't feel another one. What happens if I stop?

You have seven years to feel an emotion once the soul has released it. If you don't feel the emotion during this seven-year cycle, the next time the soul releases it, the circumstances will be harsher. This is where your 'free will' comes in. You can do whatever you want with your emotions. If you decide not to feel another emotion now, that's okay. Just know that in the future that emotion will recycle, it will come back into your life, and when it does, dealing with it will be more difficult. Preventing yourself from feeling an emotion doesn't make that emotion disappear. All it does is stuff the energy of your emotion back into your energy field. You carry that emotion with you at all times. Think of it as excess baggage. One day that suitcase is going to break open again and you will be forced to deal with it again.

6. I'm adopted and don't know my genetic patterning. How does that affect the System For Soul Memory?

Being adopted doesn't change anything. The System For Soul Memory is still the same. Because of what is written in your soul and in your genes, you attracted the adoption. To know your genetic patterning, just look at your life experiences and the emotions they brought forth during the first eight years of your life, and you will see what is written in your genes. Adoption at birth is a major Root Chakra issue and will affect how you live, work and make money. The emotion of abandonment, found in the Heart Chakra , will also be a major life issue.

7. I grew up with people who weren't my parents. How does that affect the System For Soul Memory?

Once again, like energy attracts like energy. Who ever was a major influence in your life during the first eight years will be instrumental in helping you learn your life lessons. You attracted these people by what was written in your genes. These people will have the same energy and learning lessons as your parents and your ancestors. Therefore, it doesn't affect how you use the System For Soul Memory. It does tell you though, some of your learning lessons. Not having your parents to raise you is a major abandonment issue. It will also bring up other emotions, especially those dealing with self-esteem and self-worth. Be sure to deal with those emotions.

8. **I can't remember my childhood or my seed patterns. What do I do?**

In reality, if you can't remember your childhood, it is because you are choosing *not* to remember your childhood. Fear is blocking your ability to remember. Why? What was so bad that you are hiding from it? Your subconscious remembers everything! If you want to remember, you will remember.

Once you learn how to feel an emotion fully, you should be able to remember the seed pattern, where the emotion first originated. Sometimes the memory is vague and the details are inaccurate, but the emotion will always ring true. Validating the emotions is what's most important to the soul. Also, if you speak to parents about what they remember and their version is different than yours, don't be swayed by their side of the story. They may remember the story differently. Validate your own thoughts and emotions. Don't ever let anyone talk you out of what you are feeling.

In the beginning, when you first start using the System For Soul Memory, before you become an expert at feeling your emotions, don't worry if you can't remember the seed pattern in the first eight years. An event from last year, or five years ago, or even from your teen years, will be enough to bring the emotion to the surface. Bringing the emotion to the surface, from subconscious to conscious awareness, is what is important. These events will be your seed pattern repeating itself. Logically, if you look at these events and find the similarities, you should be able to deduce what happened when you were eight and younger.

I will give you an example of how to do this. Mary can't remember her early years, yet she is positive she experienced some form of sexual abuse. She wants to remember what it was. These are the events she does remember:

A. At twelve, she was giving an oral presentation to the class when the plastic zipper on the front of her blouse separated, exposing her bare chest. The class laughed and she was mortified.

B. At twenty, she was almost date raped by a college classmate while he was driving her home from a fraternity party. He tore her blouse and fondled her breasts before she managed to get out of the car and reach safety.

C. At twenty-one she had her first experience with intercourse. Her hymen was broken and she did experience some bleeding. She enjoyed the experience and since then has had no trouble reaching orgasm.

D. At twenty-six she married. She has a good sex life with her husband, but hates it when he touches her breasts. She finds her breasts are very sensitive. She even hates to go to the gynecologist for a breast exam.

All these details of Mary's life were brought out through careful questioning. These questions were based on the two major events she could remember: what occurred at twelve and twenty. Both incidents involved her chest and breast area. Since they are repeats of what happened at a younger age, it is safe to assume that the sexual abuse she suffered in her younger years dealt with her breasts. Since she bled during her first sexual experience at twenty-one, we know she didn't experience actual rape. Another similarity between the two incidents was that they occurred in front of people she knew, but were not her family. Therefore, the abuse happened outside her home. I asked Mary to remember her date rape incident and bring up the feelings. The feeling was always of intense humiliation and shame, the same emotions suffered through every incident she remembered. When I asked her in which chakra she felt them, she pointed to the top of her head. That told us that the incident happened at the age of eight. Once we were able to deduce so many details, Mary was able to remember the incident. It did happen when she was eight. It involved her next door neighbor who was a drunk. One day, she was riding her bike past his house when he caught her and stopped her. He was very drunk, and disgusting and she could smell the alcoholic fumes. He was mumbling about how pretty she was and trying to fondle her breasts. He ripped her blouse as she managed to escape him. She rode home and hid in her room, too humiliated to tell her parents about what happened. Once she remembered the incident, Mary was able to cry and release the emotions, including how she felt about her breasts.

If you find you are struggling with an old memory, and you can't seem to bring it out, even after listing the events in your life and finding the similarities, then I always recommend seeking help. A trained hypnotherapist who can regress you back to your childhood, is a great way to bring forth a buried seed pattern.

9. The emotion I just felt was terrible. Will it be that bad again?

Once you have felt an emotion and understand that it is just energy, you will be able to feel the rest of your emotions much more easily. The more you feel, the easier it gets. Understanding the process gives you power over it. Feeling the result of how good it feels to release your emotions, then seeing the benefit of it in your life, will make you want to feel all of them.

10. Why did I begin gaining weight when I started using use the System For Soul Memory?

I find that some people begin gaining weight when they first start using the System For Soul Memory. I feel there are different reasons for this. First when you begin feeling your emotions, you are bringing more energy, more life force, into your energy field. Your subconscious doesn't know what to do with this extra energy. Sometimes your body wants to fill up the extra space with physical girth. Sometimes all this energy brings with it more emotions than you can handle. So some people store these emotions in the fat in their bodies until they can deal with them. Gaining the weight is temporary. When people begin using the System For Soul Memory, they change. Their demeanor takes on a glow. Their eyes begin to sparkle. They radiate peace, even if they are in the midst of inner turmoil. Their energy field flows smoothly and vibrantly as it was meant to.

11. Why do I get to a certain place while feeling the emotion, then stop? I can't seem to go beyond that place.

Fear is keeping you from moving forward. The fear may be caused by many different reasons. You may be afraid of experiencing more emotional pain. You may be afraid of the thoughts attached to the emotion. Maybe there are memories that will surface that you don't want to see. Your energy field and your life are also going to change once you have fully felt an emotion. Maybe you are afraid of making these changes. Some people may leave your life. You could move, change jobs. Subconsciously, you know this and won't allow yourself to accept it.

These are just some of the reasons why you won't allow the whole emotion to surface. Some people like being addicted to their misery. Are you one of them? Examine why you don't want to fully feel your emotions and you will discover the reason why.

12. My boss is the problem in my life. He triggers all these terrible feelings in me. If I change jobs won't I be leaving those bad emotions behind?

Every emotion you experience in your life is your emotion. These emotions don't come from an outside source. They come from within your soul. Everywhere you go, you carry these emotions with you. These emotions are energy and they cycle through your energy field. Your energy field walks before you and attracts similar energy fields to you. Wherever you go you keep attracting similar energy to yours. Therefore, everything in your life is a mirror of some aspect of you.

If you have a boss, or some person, who is triggering emotions in you, then you must examine whom this person represents from your childhood. This person is mirroring something that happened to you in the first eight years of your life that was emotionally painful.

If you change jobs, your energy field is still attached to you. It will continue to attract similar bosses to the one you just escaped. Like energy seeks like energy. The only way to change this is to change your energy field. And the only way to change your energy field is to feel the emotions your boss has triggered. Once you feel the emotion of what a boss like this *feels* like, you change your energy field. You will be able to spot similar bosses in the future, and avoid them. You will never be attracted to this type of person again.

13. Someone in my family is going through a terrible time. How can I help them?

When someone around you is experiencing hard times, then you know after reading this book, that this person is not dealing with an emotion that is triggering his or her crisis. You can help this person by you feeling the emotions that arise within you while you are standing in this person's presence. When you feel your emotions in his or her presence, you are sending a signal through your energy field into the other person's energy field to feel and deal with the emotions. Their subconscious will do the rest.

On a deeper level, your soul knows that everyone is God and that all energy is connected. Your emotions will be mirroring the emotions of the person you are with. When you feel your emotions in his or her presence, you are feeling his or her emotions too. Your soul knows no distinction. Therefore, you feeling your emotions helps this person heal.

18

More Techniques and Suggestions in Using the System for Soul Memory

While working with people, I discovered many helpful hints in getting people to understand the energy system of the body and how it relates to their lives. Below is a listing of these hints.

1. Generally, the people you attract into your life now will remind you of a particular aspect of one of your parents, or someone who was close to you when you were growing up. If you are currently having a problem with someone, think back to your childhood. Does this person have a similar trait or aspect to the person you grew up with? This trait is triggering the remembrance of an old hurt. The current person is reminding you of it.
2. The right side of your body is male, the left female. When doing energy work, the left hand is used to bring energy into the body. Because it is the receptive side of the body, it is considered the female side. The right hand is where energy is sent from the body to others. Because it is the achieving side, it is considered the male side. Hindu and Buddhist gurus pass *shakti*, energy, to their followers in this manner.

Therefore, if you are having a problem with a part of your body, look to see which side it's on. If it's the right side, you are having a problem with a male person in your life. If it's the left side, you are having a problem with a female. For example, Justin is a lawyer who broke his right ankle while jogging. The right side of the body is male. Ankles tend to hold old buried anger from a parent. When I asked Justin to remember what happened just before his injury, he remembered having a dispute with a client who was being irrational in taking his advice. After thinking about it, Justin realized his father was the same way. Instead of feeling the anger the client triggered, Jason tried running it off.

3. Your soul creates everything in your life. If you have an issue that seems baffling, begin thinking like your soul. Ask yourself, "Why did I create this?" If the answer doesn't immediately come to you, play a game with yourself. Make up answers. As I wrote in Chapter 15, making up answers, or being creative, frees the subconscious mind so the truth comes out. Once you have the answer, you will know how to solve the issue.
4. If one of your children is having a problem, their problem is your issue too. Your children inherit their emotions from you. They mirror them back to you. Therefore, if you work on their problem emotionally, you will be helping your child work through it. Watching your child suffer will bring up emotions in you. Feel these emotions, and validate them. Talk to your child. Ask your child what he or she is feeling. See if you can bring up his or her emotion in you. By you feeling the emotion, helps the child to feel it. This helps heal the situation. It doesn't matter whether the problem relates to illness or simple social situations, you can feel the emotions for your child.
5. If a family member or close friend is sick, you don't have to be a bystander and watch them suffer. As in the previous paragraph, the same principle of helping your child applies. If you feel the emotions their illness triggers in you, you will help them heal.

People's energy fields intermingle constantly. Your energy field affects the energy fields of those around you. What you learn on the level of the soul, you pass on through your energy field to those around you.

When you begin the process of feeling, don't be surprised at the emotions that arise within you. They may seem contradictory or irrelevant. Don't judge them, just feel them. For example, Margaret's husband had a heart attack and was near death. The emotions that surfaced seemed far-fetched, but she felt them anyway. First she felt angry with her husband for putting her through this. Then she felt hatred for him for always being so selfish and self-centered. His illness was very demanding and required all her time and attention. Finally, during the worst of the healing process, she realized how she had never accepted him for the way he was. She was always trying to change him. By the time Margaret finished feeling all her emotions, her husband's recovery was quick. Needless to say, after his recovery, their relationship was much better.

6. Your energy affects the energy of those around you. When you change your energy field by processing and releasing old buried emotions, you are asking the people around you to change their energy fields too. Like energy attracts like energy. When energies are no longer alike, they begin to repel each other.

Therefore, don't be surprised if people leave your life. Not everyone will be willing to process his or her emotions the way you did. Once your energies are not alike, you will no longer be compatible. You will no longer be comfortable being around those people. And vice-verse. They no longer will be comfortable being around you.

7. When you begin to change, don't be surprised that others get angry with you for changing. Those closest to you will feel the angriest. They will feel you changing the status quo. They may not know this consciously, but subconsciously they will

feel it. Their actions will show you they are angry. Through changing your energy field, you have disrupted and changed their energy field. Not everyone will be appreciative.

I discovered that it generally takes a year for a group to go through the changes. During that year, relationships in the group will be tough, but afterwards it will be well worth it. The whole group will be entering a new level of compatibility, love and happiness.

8. Once you feel an emotion, you change the energy of your body. Changing the energy of your body also changes it physically. This will show up in different ways.

Sometimes just after a tough emotional release you may come down with a cold or virus. This is the body's way of cleansing itself. It is taking the release of old buried emotional energy and passing it physically out the body.

You may also change physically. You may grow taller, grow bigger breasts, bigger feet, hands. Your face may change, the eye color change. It is possible for a trauma from your childhood to hinder your normal growth development. For example, the trauma of a young girl's sexual molestation could arrest the normal growth of her breasts. As an adult, after healing the old emotional wounds, her breasts may grow to their destined size.

Or the changes might be something you instigate, like desiring to cut your hair, wanting to exercise, or to lose weight. For example, maybe you were fat because your mother hounded you about your weight when you were small. Instead of feeling the hurt this caused, you acted out your feelings by eating more. Once you felt all the old hurts, you no longer created the desire to eat.

9. What is your biggest fear? Any fear stored in your subconscious is a buried, unprocessed emotion. It is caused by something that happened to you in the first eight years of your life. Eventually your soul is going to bring it to your attention. Why not think about it now and deal with it while it's still an emotion, or as I like to call it, a snowflake. If you allow the

feelings to come up now, you won't have to live them later as an avalanche.

10. If there is a competition you wish to win, there is some mental and emotional preparation you can do to assure your win. Use one of the three energy stimulators to manifest your desire. Mentally, do visualization techniques. Imagine yourself winning the competition. Then, *feel* yourself winning it.

Next, remember the rule of energy: for every action, there is an equal reaction. As soon as you create the energy of winning, you also create the energy of losing. To avoid making the energy of losing a physical reality, you can process the emotions of losing before the event. Then your soul won't make it a reality. You can do this by asking yourself why you would want to lose. Did anything happen in your childhood that would set you up to lose? Do you carry any beliefs of poor self-esteem, worthlessness, or powerlessness that could keep you from winning? If you explore and feel the emotions of losing before the event, you won't have to live the reality of losing afterwards.

11. If you have an unusual reaction to an insect bite, stop to assess why. Like energy attracts like energy. An insect is made up of energy just like you. When you attract a particular insect, you are attracting similar energy to yours. Your soul is using that insect to tell you something. Why not take a moment to assess why.

First, ask your soul why the insect came into your life. Why did it bite you? If the answer doesn't immediately come to you, don't wait for it. You'll get the answer when you least expect it.

Next, you can figure out what the insect is telling you by understanding what the insect does. For example, Cory was bitten by a mosquito and had a terrible reaction. When Cory took a moment to assess why, he was amazed at the answer. Mosquitoes are parasites. They bite you to suck off your blood. Three weeks before Cory was bitten, his mother-in-law moved in to his house. Her attitude really annoyed him. Cory felt like she was being a parasite. She took for granted his hospitality. The mosquito was trying to make Cory aware of his feelings.

12. When you begin feeling your emotions, eventually you will notice a marked improvement in your life. To gauge how you are doing in this area, answer these questions.
    Do you have everything you want? The more you feel, the more you will manifest your desires. In terms of energy, the more energy you allow to move through you without manipulation, the more energy you will attract into your life. This allows you to have all that you desire.
    Do you feel well loved? The more you love yourself, the more others will love you. Through your energy field, you are telling every one around you how to love you. If they love you well, you are allowing yourself to be well loved. If you carry any old hurts from the first eight years of your life, this will reflect in how others love you. You can gauge what emotions you still need to process, by examining how you are being loved today.
    Are you being well treated by others? How you feel about yourself is going to determine how others treat you. The more you process your emotions, the more compassion and love you will have for others. Your energy field will radiate this. People will respond in the same way. They will treat you with the same love and compassion you have for them. They will be a mirror of you. If you are being treated in a manner you don't like, look to see how you treat others. What is the old hurt that makes you act this way? For example, Georgia goes out of her way to be courteous and respectful to people. Yet when she is out in public, people are rude to her. When she stands on line waiting to be helped, she gets ignored. When she returns something to a store, she is put through the third degree and made to feel like a criminal. Georgia grew up with a critical, disapproving mother. Georgia still carries around all the old hurt. She judges her mother as being a terrible person. Georgia goes out of her way not to be like her. Yet Georgia doesn't

realize that she is being just as critical and disapproving as her mother. She doesn't realize that people are treating her the same way her mother did. Until she feels the old hurt, she won't realize this.

When you want to accomplish something, does it get done easily and without hitches? If your energy system is flowing freely, your life will flow freely. You will be able to accomplish whatever you want easily and without hassle. If you do meet with resistance, then you have an old issue that is blocking your energy field. If it is a person who is resisting you, making your life difficult, then a person from your childhood did the same thing. If it is someone in your family, then it was a family member when you were young. If it is a person who is not a part of your family, then the same applies when you were younger. If an organization or company is resisting you, making your life difficult, then an organization, school, church, or business did the same to you when you were young. If someone with authority is blocking you, then someone who had authority over you in your childhood, did the same thing. Any blocks or hitches today will mirror the blocks and hitches from your childhood.

13. If you think of each chakra as a *section of your subconscious*, governed by your soul, you will be able to understand yourself better. When you know about each chakra, then see how that chakra affects your life, you will know what lies buried in your subconscious and in your soul. You will gain a better understanding of yourself and your actions. You will gain the power to control your life.
14. If you notice that you get sick every year at the same time, then to your subconscious, that time of year marks a time when you were vulnerable. This means an emotional trauma occurred, and your subconscious is remembering it. For example, every spring Eli comes down with a terrible cold that eventually turns into pneumonia. When Eli was asked what terrible

thing happened to him in the spring, he quickly replied. When he was a young boy and living in Germany, it was the springtime when the Nazi's took him and his family to the concentration camps.

Notes

[1] "Why God Plays Dice," Mark Buchanan, *New Scientist Magazine,* August 22, 1998.

[2] *The Chakra Tapes, Mastery of Chi,* Tapes 1 and 2, Swami Paramananda Saraswatti, The Foundation for Meditative Studies, 1990.

[3] Research Guide: Aging and Genetics Fact Sheet, BioRAP, Connecticut United for Research Excellence, Inc., Copyright 1995 & 1996. <www.biorap.org> "DNA undergoes about 30 mutations during a human lifetime."

[4] Check a chart of the Central Nervous System to discover which chakra is involved. Notice where your injury lies, then follow the closest nerve ending back to the spine. That part of the spine will be sitting, in either the Root Chakra, The Navel Chakra or the Solar Plexus Chakra. Knowing the chakra will then give you a good idea of the emotional basis for your injury.

[5] Locate your injury on the chart of the central nervous system and follow the closest nerve ending back to the spine. Look at Diagram 2 to see in which chakra that part of the spine falls.

[6] *Kundalini, The Secret of Life,* Swami Muktananda, SYDA Yoga Publications, South Fallsburg, NY, 1979, p. 50.

[7] Ibid, p. 51.

[8] To find which chakra is associated with your injury, check the chart of the central nervous system as you did in the two proceeding chapters.

[9] Check the chart of the Central Nervous System to discover which chakra is involved. Notice where your injury lies, then follow the closest nerve ending back to the spine. That part of the spine will be sitting in either the Throat Chakra or the Moon Center Chakra. Knowing the chakra will then give you a good idea of the emotional basis for your injury.

[10] Check a chart of the central nervous system to discover which chakra is involved. Notice where your injury lies, then follow the closest nerve ending back to the spine. That part of the spine will be sitting in either the Throat Chakra or the Moon Center Chakra. Knowing the chakra will give you a good idea of the emotional basis for your injury.

About the Author

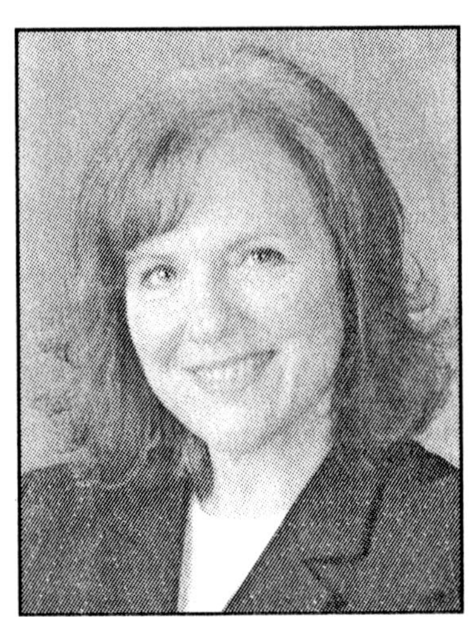

SUSAN KERR is widely known as an animal psychic and has appeared on the *Joan Rivers, Ricki Lake,* and the *Carnie Wilson Show.*

Susan obtained a Bachelors degree in Speech and Drama from Adelphi University in 1970. She spent four years studying at the Foundation for Meditative Studies in Oregon. For ten years, Ms. Kerr owned and operated StarBrite Books, a metaphysical bookstore in New York, and is a member of NAPRA. Since 1988, Ms. Kerr has been a spiritual counselor, psychic, teacher and lecturer. She regularly teaches classes on meditation, psychic development, healing and animal communication.

Susan Kerr and her husband, Michael, live in New York and share their lives with Turbo, a Bearded Collie, and Taco, a Macaw parrot. They have two adult sons, Joshua and Zachary.

Visist Susan Kerr's web site at: http://www.susankerr.com

Printed in the United States
6587